Erg AEROBICS

Why does working @ my computer hurt so much?

A comprehensive guide to help you prevent and treat
Computer Induced Repetitive Stress Injuries

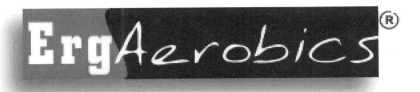

Why does working @ my computer hurt so much?

A comprehensive guide to help you prevent and treat
Computer Induced Repetitive Stress Injuries

Perry Bonomo MAPT
Daniel Seidler MSPT

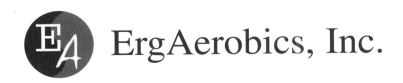

ErgAerobics, Inc.   New York

Ergle, Ergella, and Cirsi Boy are the sole property of ErgAerobics, Inc., US Trademark #s: 75/427540, 75/427541, 75/427542.

Manufactured in the United States of America
ISBN: 0-9664090-0-0
Illustrations: John Piser
Photographs: Hillary Lipstein
Page Design: Scott Metzger
Cover Design: Julie Pitman

Notice of Liability
Every precaution has been taken in the preparation of this book. Neither the authors nor ErgAerobics, Inc. shall have any liability to any person or entity with respect to any loss or damage caused or alleged to be caused directly or indirectly by the instructions contained in this book.

ErgAerobics, Inc.
24 Fifth Avenue   Suite 1222
New York, NY 10011
T. 800.689.9199   F. 530.509.9301
E-mail: info@ergaerobics.com
Web site: **www.ergaerobics.com**

Dedicated to all of our patients that have experienced CIRSIs in the past.

Table of Contents

Foreword

A generation ago the concept of ergonomics did not exist. Moreover, no one ever imagined that using a computer could lead to the kind of debilitating injuries that we see in our clinic on a daily basis.

Gregory Watchman of the Occupational Safety and Health Administration (OSHA) contends that Repetitive Stress Injuries (RSIs) "are the biggest workplace health problem in the country today." OSHA reports that RSIs account for 60% of all "workplace injuries," increasing from 27,000 in the early 1980s to 300,000 in 1993. In addition, the leading cause of illness resulting in 30 or more missed days of work is carpal tunnel syndrome, which the U.S. Department of Labor has dubbed the "occupational hazard of the 90s."

Although these statistics played a key role in our decision to study and write about Computer Induced Repetitive Stress Injuries (CIRSIs), our true inspiration for this book was our patients. They have come to us searching for relief from several kinds of CIRSIs that are a result of excessive computer use in the workplace. For example:

> The patient whose hands are so weak from carpal tunnel syndrome, which resulted from repetitive keyboarding and mouse clicking, that she can't open a bottle of soda.

> The patient whose neck hurts so much from having her monitor off to her right side that she can't even drive a car.

The secretary in our office who had such bad TMJ that she couldn't chew solid food for two weeks.

The cures for these CIRSIs are usually simple, which made us realize that we did not necessarily need to see these patients in our clinic. Their injuries should have never gotten to the point where they were in so much pain that they needed to seek professional help. So we searched for the source of their injuries and came up with this book, teaching computer users how to prevent CIRSIs.

Preventing CIRSIs is simple. Three steps are necessary.
Step 1: Properly arrange your workstation. We frequently hear descriptions of workstations that are inadvertently arranged. To us, these workstations are torture chambers. The patients we see often do not know how to properly arrange their workstations, or worse, do not even realize that their workstation set-up is the cause of their injuries.
Step 2: Sit properly at your computer. Modify your behavior to coexist more cooperatively with your computer. After all, you do spend a great deal of time with it. Shouldn't you be friends?
Step 3: Take rest breaks and perform the exercises in this book.

A good deal of our treatment in the clinic is focused on patient education. If computer users know how to set up their workstations properly (ErgArrangement), maintain good posture when sitting, and perform a few simple exercises (ErgErcises) to rejuvenate their bodies, we wouldn't hear the same stories over and over. The advice we give in this book is enough to save your career and prevent a lifetime of debilitating injuries.

To keep the material light and interesting, we created a few animated characters--Ergle, Ergella, and Cirsi Boy--to describe the causes and prevention of CIRSIs. You will read about their trials and tribulations from sitting at a computer all day. Some of their stories will remind you of problems you have encountered in your workstation.

Our goal is to have a healthier, happier computer workforce. We hope you enjoy this book and take with you a few helpful hints on how to prevent CIRSIs.

Perry and Danny

Acknowledgements

Since this project began a year and a half ago we have spoken with hundreds of people about our ideas and products. We have had many ups and downs, with things always seeming to work out in the end. We are very proud of the end results and we are extremely thankful to everyone who has helped make it possible.

Doug, Ivan, Al, and Mike @ IPS
Sheila and Debbie @ Arbon
Steve, Dave, and Ian @ Reel Life
Paul Winter
John Piser
Robin Cohen
Hayes Cohen
Robert Levin
Hillary Lipstein
Peter Scherr
Arie and Bonnie Seidler
Marcy and David Braun
Judy Swee
Louise Murphy
Michael Seidler and Mike Lehrer
Florence Dong
April Vail
David Balaban
Thomas Cuoco
Jackie Christensen
Steven and Diane

Judy and Louis Bonomo
Mark Amir
Steven Kletzkin
David Siev
Tamar Friedman
Eric Hafker
Stanley Germain

Introduction

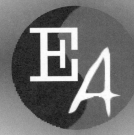

Tis better to put a strong fence 'round the top of a cliff,
Than an ambulance down in the valley.
-Joseph Malins (1895)

A white collar epidemic is sweeping our nation! According to the Department of Labor, Repetitive Stress Injuries are a **$100 billion a year** problem for corporate America. Worker's compensation costs are exorbitant and the victimized individuals often experience a lifetime of pain. ErgAerobics is a comprehensive system designed to significantly decrease your chances of experiencing Repetitive Stress Injuries.

ErgAerobics combines the latest ergonomic innovations with rehabilitation exercises designed to treat and prevent **C**omputer **I**nduced **R**epetitive **S**tress **I**njuries (**CIRSI**s). Ergonomics is the science of human interaction with machines. Adhering to some basic ergonomic principles lowers the computer user's risk of injury. Exercise increases blood flow, stretches tight muscles, and strengthens weak muscles, all of which enable the human body to be a more efficient instrument. Sound ergonomics and the right exercises can help you avoid CIRSIs for life.

ErgArrangement of your work environment is top priority before starting any job. Proper computer workstation setup is an essential step toward preventing muscle aches and pains and reducing common work fatigue. We suggest that you use ergonomic office equipment, but all of our recommendations apply to even the simplest furniture and computers. Once you properly arrange your workstation, it is imperative to position yourself correctly when working there.

Proper Posture at your workstation is an essential element in the prevention of **CIRSIs**. The most ergonomically sound computer workstation will not help you avoid injuries if you use it incorrectly. Once the workstation is set, you need to position yourself correctly within that environment. After all, you probably will be there for a while.

To prepare yourself for hours of computer use, you need to be able to tolerate the physical demands placed on you at your workstation. **ErgErcises** are exercises designed specifically to counteract the physical stresses of computer use. They are simple, inconspicuous, and time efficient. We suggest that you **ErgErcise** for **one minute each hour** when you are at work. ErgErcises will increase your endurance and overall productivity. They can be performed anytime and anywhere-- for example, during

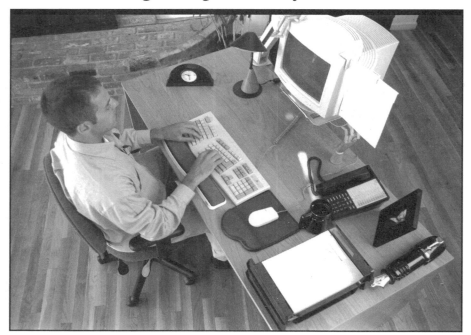

Proper ErgArrangement and sitting posture.

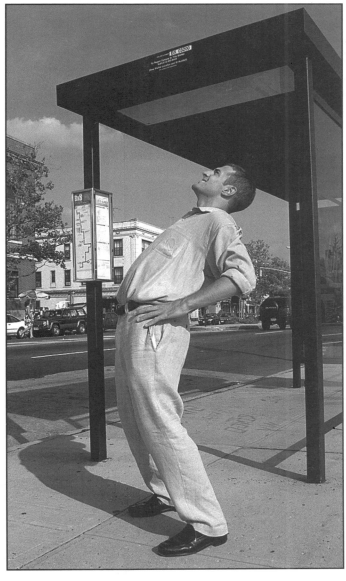

ErgErcise at the bus stop.

coffee breaks or phone conversations, or while you are waiting for the bus or train.

ErgAerobics is a comprehensive system designed to help you avoid CIRSIs and achieve excellent physical health. ErgAerobics is more than a routine--it is a way of life. Before you know it, ErgAerobics will become your ordinary way of interacting with your computer. Along with the improvement of your work habits, will come a healthier, pain-free body.

The Cast of ErgAerobics

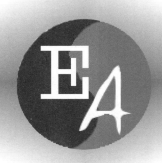

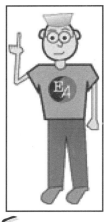

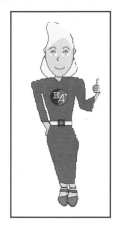

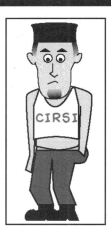

ERGLE

The eternally ergonomic star of **ErgAerobics**

ERGELLA

Ergle's love and inspiration

CIRSI BOY

Ergle's arch-enemy and the villain of **ErgAerobics**

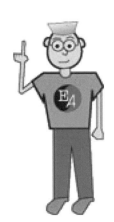

Ergle, the star of **ErgAerobics**, is a role model for all computer users. Like many of us, Ergle spends many hours a day sitting in front of his computer. Before he became the star of **ErgAerobics**, Ergle experienced the same pain that many other computer users feel after a long day of computer use. Why is sitting at a computer all day so painful? Ergle searched for answers to this question because, as a computer programmer, his livelihood was in jeopardy. The pain he felt at work affected him physically, mentally, and emotionally. One day, Ergle's soul mate and savior, Ergella, gave him a copy of **ErgAerobics**. Ergle was skeptical at first. He did not believe that this program could change his life.

One night, Ergle, defeated and tired, decided to give **ErgAerobics** a try. The exercises were easy to do, inconspicuous, and time-efficient. Ergle learned how to posture himself and set up his computer workstation properly. After a while, his pain diminished and he became more productive at work. Ergle began feeling better about himself, and his social life picked up. With his newly found confidence, Ergle finally had enough courage to ask out the object of his affection, Ergella. Of course, she said "Yes." Ergle and Ergella fell in love and recently got married.

Now that you know there is a happy ending to this story, we will describe to you, in detail, Ergle's pain before Ergella and **ErgAerobics** entered his life. We will tell you what caused Ergle's pain and how he could have avoided it.

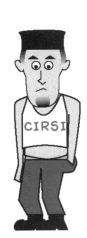

Cirsi (pronounced sir-see) **Boy** represents what Ergle once was and will never be again. Cirsi Boy and Ergle grew up together. As products of the computer age, the two boys spent many hours at their computers playing video games, doing their school work, and e-mailing friends. But Cirsi Boy was always in competition with Ergle. He had to be better at games, have better grades, and have more friends than Ergle. When they grew up, Cirsi Boy and Ergle went to the same college and took jobs at the same company.

After years of working at a computer, Cirsi Boy experienced the same pain and discomfort that Ergle did. But he refused to heed Ergella's advice and utilize the **ErgAerobics** system. Cirsi Boy's posture became more slumped, and his disposition and appearance worsened. He had fallen into the abyss of pain. As his pain increased, people found him more difficult to get along with.

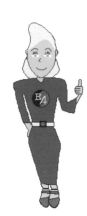

Ergella, a smart, sophisticated, ergonomically fit computer programming goddess of the '90s and beyond, is part of the minority of computer users who have never suffered from a CIRSI. Ergella has been an **ErgAerobics** follower from day one. She always works with a good posture, changing her sitting position every so often to prevent injuries. Ergella knows ErgArrangement (how to properly set up her workstation), and she takes brief rests and ErgErcise breaks to reenergize her body. As a result of this great care, her body has never "broken down" on her. Her employers love her energy and productivity, and appreciate her attempts to promote **ErgAerobics** to her coworkers. Ergella knows that her computer is not her enemy, and she wants the Cirsi Boys of the world to know that.

Why does working @ my computer hurt so much ?

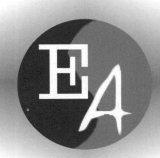

*E*rgle's work required him to sit at his computer for hours at a time. This prolonged computer use caused him lots of pain. Using his home PC didn't help his condition. As time went on, Ergle's pain increased. Ergle couldn't understand why this was happening. After all, he wasn't doing manual labor. He was just typing, maneuvering a mouse, and talking on the phone.

Ergle soon learned that his activities and the manner in which he performed them made him susceptible to microtrauma, a condition that could lead to CIRSIs. As time went on, Ergle experienced more pain because he was gradually injuring himself further. Ergle's body was eventually polluted with CIRSIs. Ergle didn't fall into the abyss of pain, he just slowly slid down the slippery slope.

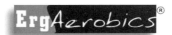

Microtrauma

- Microtrauma is the gradual wear and tear on the body from everyday activities.
- Most injuries that occur at a computer work station are the result of cumulative microtrauma.
- Microtrauma does not occur suddenly like a broken arm or leg (known as macrotrauma).
- Increased workload on active muscles requires increased blood flow. The necessary blood flow is jeopardized by poor posture.
- It may take several months or years of poor posture and performance of a repetitive motion before you feel any pain.
- Pain can occur in the following forms:

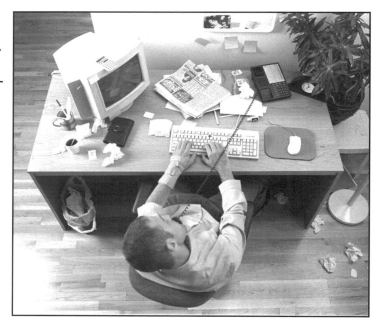

Poor ErgArrangement and sitting posture.

  - Burning
  - Aching
  - Stabbing
  - Shooting
  - Tingling
- These pains can easily be prevented by taking the following steps:
  1. ErgErcise--Performing preventative stretching and strengthening exercises.
  2. Maintaining good posture throughout the day.
  3. Correcting computer workstation ErgArrangement.
  4. Taking regular rest breaks.

Repetitive Stress Injuries (RSIs) & Computer Induced Repetitive Stress Injuries (CIRSIs)

- An RSI is any injury caused by a repetitive activity.
- RSIs result from cumulative microtrauma.
- CIRSIs are any RSIs that result from the cumulative microtraumas caused by the repetitive activities associated with using a computer. It is difficult to eliminate many of these activities.

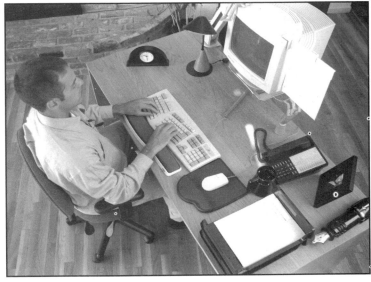

Repetitive activity at a computer

- Good posture makes a computer user less susceptible to CIRSIs by enabling blood to flow to the necessary muscles.
- Periodic breaks, in addition to stretching and strengthening ErgErcises, accomplish the following:
  - Increase blood flow to working muscles.
  - Remove irritating waste products from overworked muscles.
  - Reduce fatigue.
  - Improve overall efficiency and effectiveness at work.

Ergella's ErgArrangement Checklist

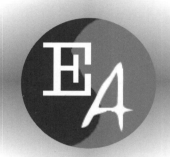

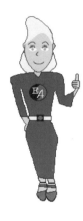

Computer Set-Up

Desk:

- ☐ Large enough to hold the keyboard, mouse, monitor, and documents
- ☐ Rounded edges.

Monitor:

- ☐ Top edge at eye level or less than 6 inches below.
- ☐ Ability to tilt vertically and horizontally.
- ☐ Monitor and document holder directly in front of user, not off to either side.
- ☐ Approximately arms' length from the user.
- ☐ To reduce glare, position monitor so that it is perpendicular to any windows and not directly beneath overhead lights.

Keyboard and mouse:

☐ Keyboard and mouse pads to maintain wrists in neutral position (not bent up, down, in, or out).

☐ Split keyboard for more ergonomic wrist and arm positioning.

☐ Rounded edges on keyboard to soften the areas of contact for your wrists and hands.

Chair:

☐ Separately adjustable back and seat cushions.

☐ Adjustable, padded arm rests.

☐ Lumbar support pad or roll.

☐ Padded seat with slight hollow to prevent sliding.

☐ Ability to swivel for accessibility to unreachable objects.

☐ Five castor wheels for mobility and stability.

☐ Adequate space beneath chair and desk to bend and straighten knees comfortably.

☐ Footrest, if feet don't rest flat on the ground.

User Positioning:

Note: All of the equipment we recommend has adjustment capabilities that allow you to achieve the following positioning:

• Sit down in your chair with your arms on the armrests.

• If you don't have armrests, push your keyboard and mouse back far enough to rest your forearms on your desk.

• Place your feet flat on the floor or get support from a footrest.

• Raise or lower your chair so that your knees are at an angle just greater than 90° (hips higher than knees).

- Slightly arch your lower back with the support of a lumbar cushion or pillow.
- Spread your upper back into the back of the chair.
- Move your head back to align with your spine so that your ears are directly over your shoulders and hips.

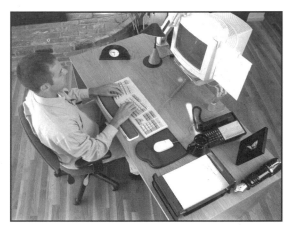

ErgArrangement

- Tuck your chin down slightly so that your eyes are looking straight ahead at the center of your monitor.
- Rest your arms comfortably at your sides.
- Bring your shoulders directly above your hips.
- Rest your forearms on padded armrests at the height that:
    - Your wrists are a little bit lower than your elbows.
    - Your elbows are bent and about an inch in front of your trunk.
    - Your wrists are in a neutral position (not bent upward or downward).

ERGLETIP: TAKE A DEEP BREATH AND RELAX.

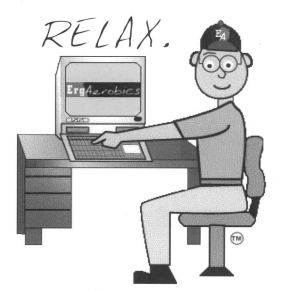

Stretching and Strengthening

E4

*E*rgle always tried to keep himself in shape. When he was in high school, he played varsity tennis and golf. When he went off to college, he worked out at the gym three times a week. He thought this was enough to keep him physically fit. But as his college courses got harder, Ergle's workload at the computer increased and he began feeling the aches and pains associated with sitting at a computer all day. At the time, Ergle did not realize that periodic stretching and strengthening breaks could have helped him prevent CIRSIs and promote his well being.

ERGELLATIP: BEFORE PERFORMING ANY OF THE FOLLOWING ERGERCISES, IT IS RECOMMENDED THAT YOU FIRST READ THE BACKGROUND INFORMATION ON STRETCHING AND STRENGTHENING.

Stretching

- Stretching is a key component to any workout program.
- Before starting any exercise, it is important to warm up the muscles and prepare them for the activities by stretching.
- Many injuries can occur if the muscles aren't warmed up and properly stretched.
- Many people stretch incorrectly, causing them to do more harm than good.
- It is important to understand when, why, and how to stretch.

When to Stretch

- After a brief warm-up and at the end of a workout. Stretching is easier at the end of a workout because your muscles are fatigued and relaxed. Stretching at the end of a workout also helps to prevent lactic acid accumulation, which can lead to muscle soreness.
- In the morning, before you start your day. Your muscles are usually tighter in the morning than they are in the evening.
- At work, after sitting or standing for long periods of time.
- Any time during the day when you are watching television, listening to music, or talking on the phone. Stretching is easy and time-efficient.
- You do not need expensive equipment, just proper technique.

Why Stretch

- Reduces muscle tension, enabling the body to relax.
- Promotes greater flexibility.
- Prevents injuries. (A tight muscle has a greater chance of being strained than a loose muscle does.)

- Allows easy and free movement.
- Promotes circulation.
- Sends signals to your muscles that they are about to work.

How to Stretch

- Stretch until you feel a slight discomfort and then relax.
- Stretching should not be painful. If it is, then you are overdoing it.
- Try to hold your stretch for 10-20 seconds.
- Breathe slowly and deeply when stretching. This should help you relax and give you a better stretch.
- Focus on the area being stretched.
- Do not bounce or jerk when stretching. Stretching should be performed in a smooth, steady fashion. Bouncing actually tightens the muscle you are trying to stretch.
- Always stretch within your own limits. Do not compare yourself to others and try to stretch more.

Strengthening

- Strengthening muscles has many benefits for a computer user.
  - Strong muscles are less likely to fatigue, resulting in greater productivity throughout the work day.
  - The chance for muscle breakdown during work decreases along with the likelihood for injuring oneself.
- There are many simple, effective strengthening exercises you can perform at your workstation.
- It is important for the computer user to understand how to strengthen muscles properly, when to perform these exercises, and why

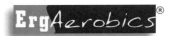

strengthening exercises are beneficial.
- These exercises do not involve weights, just know-how.

When to Strengthen

- For best results, strengthen each section of your body 1-3 times per week.
- Strengthen after a brief warm-up and stretch to awaken your muscles.
- Perform strengthening exercises any time you have a free moment during the day.

Why Strengthen

- Increases the strength and endurance of your muscles.
- Prevents injuries.
- Increases productivity throughout the work day.
- Promotes circulation.
- Strong postural muscles allow you to maintain proper posture for prolonged periods of time.

How to Strengthen

- All exercises should be done in a slow, controlled manner.
- Be consistent. Stay on a regular schedule throughout the workday and workweek.
- Forget all about "No Pain, No Gain." Any strengthening exercise that causes pain should be discontinued or modified.

Posture: More than "Sit up straight."

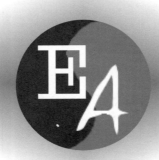

*A*s a youngster, Ergle was always told by his parents and teachers to sit up straight. Ergle was a good kid and he usually tried to heed this advice. But as time went by, he began having difficulty sitting up straight while working at his computer. It should be noted that no one ever showed Ergle how to maintain good posture at a computer workstation.

Ergle developed a Slouched Sitting Posture, Forward Head Posture, and Rounded Shoulders. These poor postural habits decreased Ergle's ability to work effectively at his computer and eventually contributed to CIRSIs.

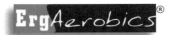

The Importance of Posture

ErgIeFact: The way you posture your entire body while working at a computer is vital to preventing neck, arm, leg, and back CIRSIs.

GOOD POSTURE

↓

Provides adequate blood supply to and from muscles.

↙   ↘

Removes irritating waste products (lactic acid) from muscles and the body.

Brings necessary vitamins and minerals to repair muscles.

↓   ↓

Prevents Repetitive Stress Injuries.

Helps muscles work effectively.

↓   ↓

Energizes your body to work more effectively.

Good Posture

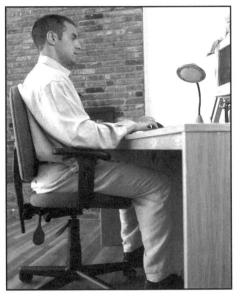

Good sitting posture

- When sitting at a computer workstation, always try to sit an inch taller than you normally do.
- Align your ears directly over your shoulders.
- Align your shoulders directly over your hips.
- Position your head evenly between both shoulders. Do not tilt your head in one direction or the other.
- When looking down, your head should be positioned over your neck and not in front of your shoulders.
- For a more detailed description, see the chapter on computer workstation ErgArrangement.

Poor Posture

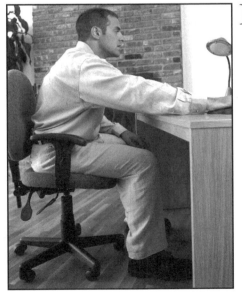

Poor sitting posture

I. Slouched Sitting Posture

A. Forces the liquid matter from your lower back discs toward the back of the spine, potentially causing a Herniated Lower Back Disc.

B. Multiplies the already stressful forces placed on your entire spine while you are sitting.

C. Over-stretches the postural muscles that support your spine.

D. Can cause:
1. Carpal Tunnel Syndrome
2. Lower Back Pain
3. Neck Pain.

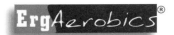

II. Forward Head Posture

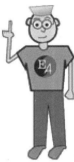

ErgleFact: Forward Head Posture can cause your head to exert 3 times more force than normal on the postural muscles in the back and sides of your neck.

A. Occurs when your head and ears are positioned in front of your shoulders, not directly over them.

B. Causes the muscles at the base of your head and neck to tighten, restricting blood flow through your head, neck, and arms.

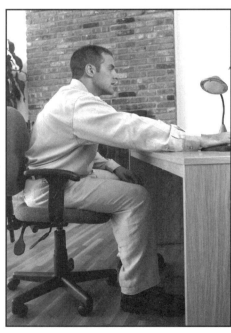

Forward Head Posture

C. Causes the muscles at the base of your head and neck to tighten, pressing on nerves. This can cause headaches and neck pain. Potentially, pain can shoot down your arms to your hands.

D. Computer users often strain to see their monitor, causing them to sit with a Forward Head Posture.

E. Once sitting with Forward Head Posture, it is necessary to tip your head back in order to see something directly in front of you. This is a potentially harmful postural position.

F. Can cause:

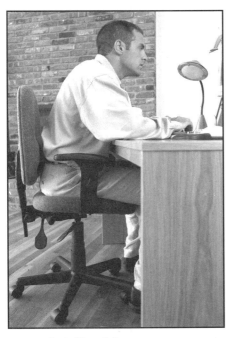

Rounded Shoulders

1. Carpal Tunnel Syndrome
2. Cervical Disc Herniation
3. Thoracic Outlet Syndrome
4. TMJ Dysfunction.

III. Rounded Shoulders

A. Occurs when your shoulders are not aligned directly over your hips and directly below your ears.

B. Causes undue stress on the shoulder tendons and subsequent tightening of the upper arm muscles.

C. Can cause:

1. Carpal Tunnel Syndrome
2. Shoulder Impingement Syndrome.

Sitting Posture

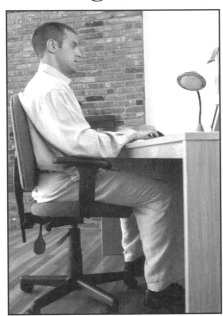

Good Sitting Posture

• When sitting, your lumbar spine is in a flexed position.

• Sitting is one of the worst stresses for your lower back.

• Sitting puts constant pressure on the front of your lower back discs, forcing the fluid backwards. This can eventually cause a Herniated Lower Back Disc.

• When sitting for long periods every day, even perfect sitting posture will not save you from eventual neck or back pain.

• Take breaks. Stand up. Perform a Skywatcher

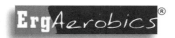

ErgErcise. This will reverse the pressure on your lumbar discs, by pushing the disc fluid forward.

Sustained Posture

- Maintaining the same posture for long periods of time requires the postural muscles to work constantly without a rest.
- Without sufficient rest or change of posture, irritating waste products accumulate in the postural muscles.
- Adequate blood flow is necessary to remove irritating waste products and refuel the postural muscles.
- Even perfect posture, if sustained for long periods of time, limits blood flow.
- Changing your posture every half hour, even slightly, shifts the stress to different postural muscles, allowing others to rest and refuel.
- Options for postural changes:
    1. Slightly raise or lower your chair.
    2. Move your lumbar pillow up or down.
    3. Stand up.
    4. Move closer to or further from your desk.
    5. Raise or lower your armrests, keyboard stand, or desk.

Postural muscles

- Muscles in your back, neck, and stomach regions which help you sit and stand erect.
- They must receive enough blood supply to maintain your head upright and your back straight throughout the day.
- The function of these muscles is to sustain your posture for long periods of time.

- Having strong postural muscles will help you maintain good posture for longer periods of time. This leads to greater productivity at work.
- Postural ErgErcises will help you achieve this.

Postural ErgErcises

Egyptian

<u>Position:</u> **Sitting or Standing**

1. Look straight ahead, not up or down.
2. Press your chin with your index finger.
3. Glide your head back on your neck making a "double chin."

<u>Hold position for:</u> **5 seconds**

<u>Repetitions:</u> **10 times.**

<u>Purpose:</u>

- Strengthens the postural muscles in the back of the neck.
- Stretches muscles around the neck.
- Prevents:
    - Forward Head Posture.
    - Cervical Disc Herniation.
    - Thoracic Outlet Syndrome.
    - TMJ Dysfunction.
    - Carpal Tunnel Syndrome.

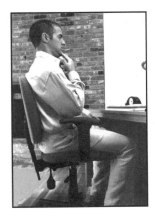

Egyptian

Tough Guy

<u>Position:</u> **Sitting or Standing**

1. Bring your shoulders back.
2. Pinch your shoulder blades together.

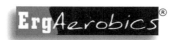

Hold position for: **5 seconds**

Repetitions: **10 times**

Purpose:

- Strengthens the rhomboids (postural muscles in the back of the shoulders and the upper back).
- Prevents
    - Rounded Shoulders.
    - Pain in the upper back and shoulders.
    - Pain, tingling, and numbness from shooting all the way down the arms.
    - Shoulder Impingement.

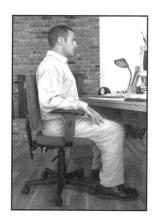

Tough Guy

Frankenstein

Position: **Sitting or Standing**

1. Let your arms hang down by your sides.
2. Shrug your shoulders up.

Hold position for: **5 seconds**

Repetitions: **10 times**

Purpose:

- Strengthens the upper trapezius (muscles which elevate the shoulders and support the head).
- Prevents:
    - Rounded Shoulders.
    - Pain in the neck, upper back, and shoulders.
    - Pain, tingling, and numbness from shooting all the way down the arms.

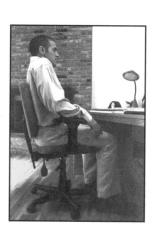

Frankenstein

Genie

<u>Position:</u> **Sitting or Standing**

1. Cross your arms over your chest.
2. Lift your elbows up to shoulder height, keeping your arms crossed.
3. Pull your arms back, pinching your shoulder blades together.

<u>Hold position for:</u> **5 seconds**

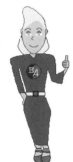

ERGELLATIP: REGARDLESS OF WHAT POSITION YOU SLEEP IN, YOUR NECK SHOULD BE STRAIGHT. YOUR HEAD SHOULD NOT BE BENT TO EITHER SIDE OR TOO FAR FORWARD OR BACK. FOR MOST PEOPLE THIS MEANS USING 1 OR 2 PILLOWS.

<u>Repetitions:</u> **5 times**

<u>Purpose:</u>

- Strengthens the rhomboids (postural muscles in the back of the shoulders and the upper back).
- Prevents:
  - Rounded Shoulders.
  - Pain in the upper back and shoulders.
  - Pain, tingling, and numbness from shooting all the way down the arms.

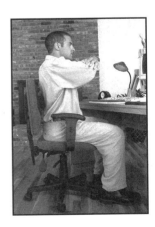

Genie

The BACKground

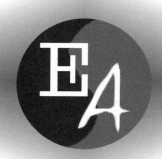

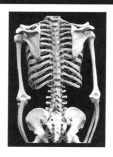 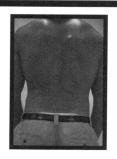 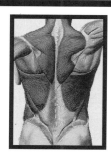

*O*ne morning, Ergle stepped out of his house, bent down to pick up his newspaper and it happened! Pain! From the right side of his lower back, down the outside of his right leg, and into the toes of his right foot. How, Ergle wondered, could this happen from just bending forward? After all, he did this every morning and never felt pain before.

From the time Ergle was in grade school, through high school and college, he spent many hours a day sitting. He sat in class, he sat when he ate, and he sat at his computer while doing homework and playing games. Once he starting working, Ergle sat for even longer periods of time throughout the *day. Because Ergle was not well versed on basic ergonomic principles, his years of improper sitting began taking a toll on his lower back discs. Gradually, the discs got weaker until that ill-fated morning when he bent over and felt pain. Ergle had Herniated a Lower Back Disc, which pressed on the nerves that ran down his lower back, sending pain through his legs to his toes. Ergle's Herniated Lower Back Disc caused him great pain for the next two months. He vowed to avoid a reoccurrence, however possible.*

The Lower Back Region

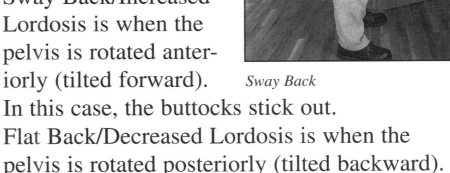

- There are five lower back vertebrae, each separated by shock absorbent discs.
- Nerves exiting the spinal cord in the lower back region travel all the way to the tips of the toes.
- The curve in the lower back is called the lumbar lordosis.

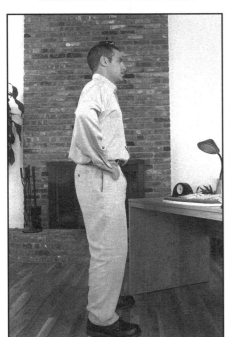

Flat Back

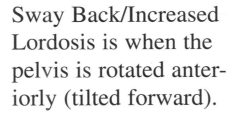

Sway Back

- Sway Back/Increased Lordosis is when the pelvis is rotated anteriorly (tilted forward). In this case, the buttocks stick out.
- Flat Back/Decreased Lordosis is when the pelvis is rotated posteriorly (tilted backward). In this case the buttocks are tucked in.
- The muscles that attach anteriorly and posteriorly to the pelvis play a major role in maintaining a proper lordosis in the spine.
- Sway Back is often caused by the hip flexor muscles (iliopsoas and rectus femoris), which

47

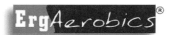

run from the front of the spine and pelvis to the front of the knee. When these muscles are tight, they pull the pelvis forward (anteriorly), increasing lordosis.

- Flat Back is often caused by the hamstring muscles, which run from the back of the knee to the back of the pelvis. When these muscles are tight they pull the pelvis back (posteriorly), reducing lordosis.
- Maintaining the proper lumbar lordosis will help you keep your lower back healthy.

How do your discs work?

- Think of a disc as a balloon with water inside of it.
- If you place a balloon on a flat surface and press on one side of the balloon, you will notice that the water inside moves to the other side.
- The gel inside your discs reacts in the same manner as water inside of a balloon.
- If you are constantly leaning forward, you are putting pressure on the front of the discs, forcing the gel to be pushed to the back.

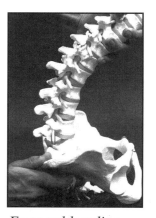

Forward bending

- If you are constantly leaning backward, you are putting pressure on the back of the discs, forcing the gel to be pushed to the front.
- If you lean toward the right, the gel goes to the left and if you lean toward the left, the gel goes to the right.
- If water inside a balloon is constantly pushed toward one side, the balloon might break, causing the water to burst out of the balloon. The same holds true for your discs.

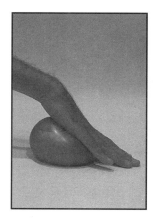

Disc reaction to forward bending

- A "bulging disc" occurs when the gelatinous substance inside is pushed in one direction. This causes a bulge in one side of the disc, but does not cause the gelatinous substance to break through the outer covering that supports the disc.
- A "herniated disc" occurs when the gelatinous substance breaks through the outer covering.
- Either a "herniated" or "bulging" disc can cause pressure to be placed on an adjacent nerve root, which will cause subsequent pain and numbness. But there are known cases of people with herniated and/or bulging discs who experience no pain. This is because the bulge or herniation is not pressing on a nerve root.

Note: If you are currently feeling pain in your lower back, stand up from your computer and roll your pelvis anteriorly (forward), and posteriorly (backward), trying to find the most comfortable and pain free position for your pelvis. Once you find that position, try to maintain it throughout the day. If you are not used to this posture, you might experience muscle soreness, so do not be alarmed. This new posture might feel awkward to you at first, but stick with it.

What is causing your Lower Back Pain?

Herniated Lower Back Disc

- A Herniated Lower Back Disc occurs when the gelatinous fluid within a lower back disc escapes the outer coating of the disc.
- A herniation can occur to the left, right, front, or back of a disc.
- Most discs herniate toward the back because people perform most of their daily activities in a forward flexed posture at the waist. This causes the gel inside the discs to be pushed backward.
- If pushed far enough backward, a disc will exceed its ordinary boundaries and pinch a nearby nerve, causing pain.
- When a Herniated Lower Back Disc pinches a lower back nerve, you could feel pain all the way down to your toes. This is due to the fact that nerves originating in your lower back run all the way down your toes.

Facet Joint Pain

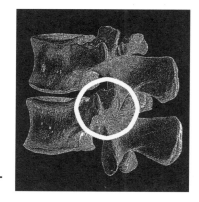

- Sway Back/Increased Lordosis causes the facet joints of adjoining vertebrae to be closer in proximity than they normally are.
- This closer proximity creates a decreased joint space, prohibiting normal motion at these usually flexible joints.

Facet Joint between two lumbar vertebrae

- The close proximity of the facet joints in someone with a Sway Back prohibits backward bending of the spine.
- Flexibility can be decreased to the point that facet joints get jammed.
- Jamming of facet joints can potentially cause inflammation, with subsequent pinching of the nerves exiting the spinal column.

Muscle Spasm

1. Poor posture
2. Sedentary posture for long periods of time
3. Repetitive activities

↓

Decreased blood flow to muscles.

↙ ↘

Waste products (lactic acid) not being flushed from working muscles.

Decreased supply of fuel necessary for muscles to work.

↘ ↙

Muscles unable to work effectively begin to shake, gasping for fuel.

↓

MUSCLE SPASM!!!

ERGLEFACT: STOP YOUR ACTIVITY. A MUSCLE SPASM IS A WARNING TO YOU THAT A GREATER INJURY IS ABOUT TO OCCUR IF THE STRESSES CURRENTLY PLACED ON YOUR BODY ARE NOT REDUCED.

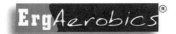

Symptoms of Lower Back Pain

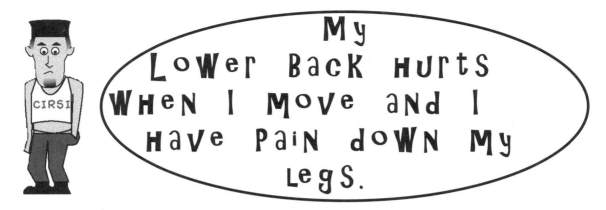

- Pain in one or both sides of the lower back.
- Pain in one or both buttocks or legs.
- The following symptoms can occur in one or both legs and potentially radiate all the way down to the toes:
    - Tingling
    - Numbness
    - Weakness.

> *Note: The above Lower Back Pain symptoms occur when a person experiences a Herniated Lumbar Disc, Facet Joint Pain, or a Muscle Spasm.*

Who is @ risk for Lower Back Pain?

- People with a poor sitting posture.
- Sedentary workers have an incidence rate of Lower Back Pain equal to that of heavy laborers.
- Many people who experience Lower Back Pain cannot attribute the pain to a specific cause.

- Risk increases at age 25 and peaks between the ages of 40 and 45.
- Men and women are equally at risk.

ERGLEFACT: 80% OF ALL PEOPLE EXPERIENCE LOWER BACK PAIN FOR A WEEK OR LONGER AT LEAST ONCE IN THEIR LIVES.

Treatment of Lower Back Pain: Getting Better

- ErgErcises to stretch and strengthen back, trunk, and leg muscles.
- Workstation ErgArrangement to minimize work-related stress to the lower back.
- Avoid or, at least, minimize painful activities.
- Improve posture to eliminate lower back stress.
- Apply ice to the region for 10-minute intervals, 3 to 5 times per day, for the first 48 hours after experiencing pain.
- Massage the area to flush out irritating waste products.
- Modalities, such as electric stimulation and ultrasound, administered by a Physical Therapist.

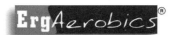

> *Note: Lower Back Pain is often not attributed to a specific anatomical structure; therefore, health practitioners often treat Lower Back Pain with the goal of achieving overall improved spinal health. The goal of ErgAerobics is to help you maintain or improve your spinal health before you have an incident of Lower Back Pain.*

Avoid Lower Back Pain: Prevention

- Workstation ErgArrangement to minimize work-related stress to the lower back.
- ErgErcises to stretch and strengthen the lower back muscles.
- Take regular breaks from the mouse and keyboard.
- Proper posture. This includes modifying your posture about twice per hour.
- Use of a lumbar roll whenever seated.
- Use of proper body mechanics, especially when bending forward.

Lower Back ErgErcises

I. Warm Up
Sky Watcher

Position: **Standing**

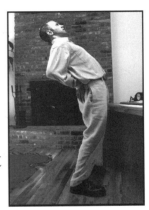

1. Place your feet shoulders' width apart.
2. Place each of your hands on your buttocks, as if you were putting them in your back pockets.
3. Slowly lean backward until you feel a slight pull in your back.
4. Keep your chin tucked into your chest and look up at the sky (or ceiling).
5. Return to the starting position.

Repetitions: **10 times**

Sky Watcher

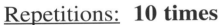

ERGLETIP: IF THIS IS A PAIN-FREE MOVEMENT FOR YOU, YOU SHOULD PERFORM THIS ERGERCISE EVERY TIME YOU STAND UP.

Purpose:
- Increases blood flow into the lower back muscles.
- Reverses the stresses of sitting with a forward flexed posture.
- Stretches the flexor muscles of the lower back.
- Prevents Lower Back Pain.

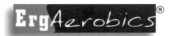

II. Stretch
Toe Kiss

Position: **Sitting**

1. Slide your chair back from your desk.
2. Move your buttocks toward the front of your desk chair.
3. Place your feet firmly on the ground.
4. Place your hands on your knees and slowly slide them down your shins until you feel a slight pull in your lower back.

Hold position for: **10 seconds**

5. Slide your hands back up to your knees and slowly push yourself up to the starting position.

Repetitions: **5 times**

ERGLETIP: FOR AN ADDED STRETCH, TAKE DEEP BREATHS INTO YOUR ABDOMEN WHILE STILL IN THIS POSITION.

Purpose:
- Stretches the extensor muscles of the lower back.
- Increases blood flow into the lower back muscles.
- Relaxes the lower back muscles by relieving stress and tension.
- Prevents Lower Back Pain.

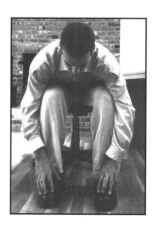

Toe Kiss

Who's There?

<u>Position:</u> **Sitting**

1. Keep your feet flat on the ground or on a footrest.
2. Slowly reach with your left hand to your right armrest while twisting at the waist.
3. Take deep breaths throughout the movement.

<u>Hold position for:</u> **10 seconds**

4. Slowly reach with your right hand to your left armrest while twisting at the waist.
5. Take deep breaths.

<u>Repetitions:</u> **5 times in each direction, alternating left and right**

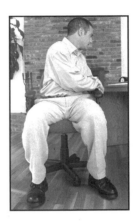

Who's There?

<u>Purpose:</u>
- Stretches the muscles on either side of your waist.
- Increases blood flow into the lower back muscles.
- Relaxes the lower back muscles by relieving stress and tension.
- Prevents Lower Back Pain.

Wheel Touch

<u>Position:</u> **Sitting**

1. Place both of your feet flat on the ground or on a footrest.
2. Let your arms hang straight down along the outside of your armrests.
3. Slowly bend your torso over your left armrest, reaching toward the ground with your left hand.

<u>Hold position for:</u> **10 seconds**

4. Slowly return to the starting position.

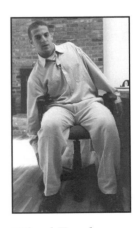

Wheel Touch

5. Slowly bend your torso over your right armrest, reaching toward the ground with your right hand.

<u>Repetitions:</u> **5 times**

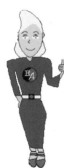

ERGELLATIP: DO NOT REACH TOO FAR. IT IS EASY TO LOSE YOUR BALANCE IF YOUR CHAIR IS NOT STURDY. IT IS NOT IMPORTANT THAT YOU ACTUALLY REACH THE GROUND. YOU SHOULD JUST FEEL A SLIGHT PULL ON THE OPPOSITE SIDE OF WHICH YOU ARE REACHING.

<u>Purpose:</u>
- Stretches the abdominal obliques and quadratus lumborum (muscles on either side of the waist).
- Increases blood flow into the lower back muscles.
- Relaxes the lower back muscles by relieving stress and tension.
- Prevents Lower Back Pain.

The Thinker

<u>Position:</u> **Sitting**
1. Place both of your feet flat on the ground.
2. Lift your left foot up and place it on your right knee.
3. Lean forward slowly, being careful not to lose your balance.

<u>Hold position for:</u> **10 seconds**

<u>Repetitions:</u> **5 times**

4. Repeat with your right foot on your left knee.

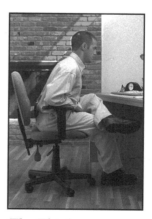

The Thinker

Purpose:
- Stretches the piriformis and gluteals (muscles of the buttock and back of the upper leg).
- Increases blood flow into the buttocks and the legs.
- Reduces muscle tension in the buttocks and legs.
- Prevents Lower Back Pain.

Hamstring Stretch

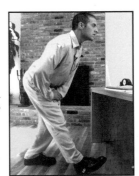

Position: **Standing**
1. Place your right foot one step length in front of you.
2. Slowly bend forward at the waist.
3. Place both of your hands on your right knee, keeping that knee straight.
4. Point the toes of your right foot towards the ceiling.

Hold position for: **10 seconds**

Hamstring Stretch

Repetitions: **5 times**
5. Place your left foot one step length in front of you.
6. Repeat with your left leg.

Purpose:
- Stretches the hamstrings (muscles in the back of your upper leg and down to the back of your knee). Hamstring flexibility is very important for the maintenance of proper posture.
- Reduces muscle tension in the back of the legs.
- Increases circulation in the legs.
- Prevents Lower Back Pain.

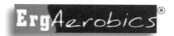

III. Strengthen

Briefcase Lift

<u>Position:</u> **Sitting**

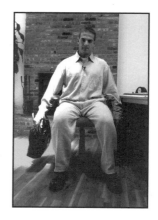

1. Place both of your feet flat on the ground or on a footrest.
2. Get a medium-weight object to hold in your left hand. Start with a book. Over several weeks, work your way up to your briefcase.
3. Let your left arm hang outside your left armrest.

Briefcase Lift

4. With your left arm, book in hand, slowly bend over your left armrest.
5. Bend until you feel a slight pull on your right side.
6. Slowly come up.

<u>Repetitions:</u> **10 times**

7. Switch the object to your right hand and repeat the action on your right side.

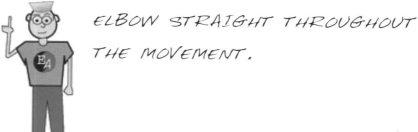

ErgleTip: BE SURE TO KEEP YOUR ELBOW STRAIGHT THROUGHOUT THE MOVEMENT.

<u>Purpose:</u>

- Strengthens the abdominal oblique and quadratus lumborum (muscles on either side of the waist).
- Stabilizes the lower back.
- Prevents Lower Back Pain.

Pillow Squeeze

<u>Position:</u> **Sitting**

1. Place your arms on your armrests or in your lap.
2. Place your feet flat on the floor or on a footrest.
3. Press your lower back into your lumbar pillow or chairback.

<u>Hold position for:</u> **5 seconds**

<u>Repetitions:</u> **10 times**

<u>Purpose:</u>

- Strengthens the lower abdominal muscles.
- Stabilizes the lower back.
- Prevents Lower Back Pain.

Resistance March

<u>Position:</u> **Sitting**

1. Place both of your feet flat on the floor.
2. Lift your left knee toward the ceiling until your foot is 6 inches from the ground.
3. With your foot raised, press down on the top of your knee with the palm of your left hand.
4. Do not allow your foot to be pushed down.

<u>Hold position for:</u> **5 seconds**

<u>Repetitions:</u> **5 times**

5. Repeat with your right leg, resisting with your right hand.

<u>Purpose:</u>

- Strengthens the lower abdominal and lower back muscles.
- Strengthens the hip flexors (muscles of the upper

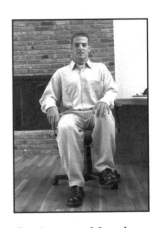

Resistance March (left)

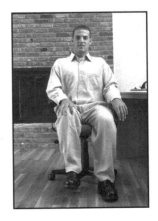

Resistance March (right)

61

leg).
- Stabilizes the lower back.
- Prevents Lower Back Pain.

Up to your NECK

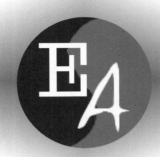

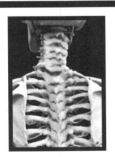 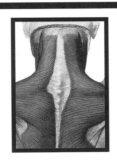 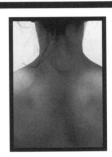

*E*rgle has always had a lot of friends. Although he would always be working at his computer, Ergle frequently talked on the phone while typing. Ergle needed his hands to type so he used his head and shoulders to support the phone. Ergle's head would be tilted towards one side for many hours at a time. Little did he know, but this posture caused his muscles to tighten and the disc fluid in his neck to be pushed in one direction. Our poor Ergle was in pain again. He felt pain on the left side of his neck and a shooting pain down his left arm.

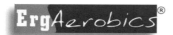

The Cervical Region

- There are 7 cervical (neck) vertebrae, each separated by shock absorbing discs.
- The discs allow for free movement of the vertebrae in all directions.
- Nerves exiting the spinal cord in the neck region continue all the way to the tips of the fingers.
- The natural curve in your neck is called your cervical lordosis.
- The postural muscles of the neck help maintain your cervical lordosis and support your head in the upright position. Several main arteries pass through this region in order to reach the arms and hands.
- Any tightening of the postural muscles of the neck, chest and shoulder can seriously inhibit blood flow and/or nerve conduction to the arm and hand. This can cause pain, tingling and numbness throughout the entire arm and hand.

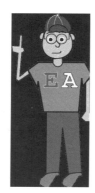 PLEASE REFER TO "HOW DO YOUR DISCS WORK?" FOR MORE DETAILED INFORMATION.

What is causing your Neck Pain?

Herniated Cervical Disc

- A Herniated Cervical Disc occurs when the gelatinous fluid within a neck disc escapes the outer coating of the disc. Continuous repeated movements or sustained posture can cause this to happen over time.

- Most discs herniate towards the back because people perform most of their daily activities with a Forward Head Posture, causing the fluid inside the discs to be pushed backwards.
- A herniation can also occur to the left, right, or forward.
- If pushed far enough, a disc will exceed its ordinary boundaries and pinch a nearby nerve, causing pain.
- Generally, the nerves originating in your neck run down your arms.
- A nerve in your neck being pinched by a Herniated Cervical Disc can possibly cause pain all the way down to your fingers. This is due to the fact that nerves originating in your neck run through your arms.

Thoracic Outlet Syndrome

- The thoracic outlet is an area in the side of the neck that 5 major nerves and 2 main arteries pass through in order to reach the arms and hands.

ERGLEFACT: THORACIC OUTLET SYNDROME OFTEN CAUSES YOU TO WAKE UP WITH A DEAD ARM.

- Any tightening of the postural muscles of the neck, chest and shoulder can seriously inhibit blood flow and/or nerve conduction to the arm and hand. This can cause pain, tingling and numbness throughout the entire arm and hand.

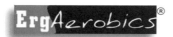

Symptoms of Neck Pain

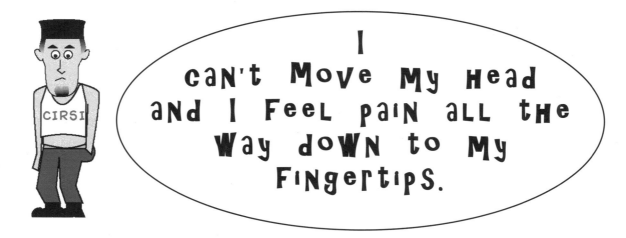

> Note: The following symptoms occur due to both of the above neck injuries, Cervical Disc Herniation and Thoracic Outlet Syndrome.

- Pain, tingling and numbness anywhere from the neck to the hand.
- Skin changes of the neck, arm, and hand.
- Weakness of the muscles in the neck, arm, and hand.

Who is @ risk for Neck Pain?

- Computer workers with poor posture or sustained posture.
- People engaged in overhead activities, i.e. filing, painting.
- People typing at a computer with their arms unsupported.
- Telephone users who constantly tilt their head to one side.
- People who sleep with too many pillows.

Treatment of Neck Pain: Getting Better

- ErgErcises to stretch and strengthen the muscles of the neck and shoulder regions.
- Workstation ErgArrangement to minimize work stresses to the neck region.
- Avoid, or at least, minimize painful activities.
- Postural improvement to prevent Forward Head Posture.
- Ice the neck region for 10 minute intervals, 3-5 times per day for the first 48 hours after first experiencing pain.
- Massage in order to flush irritating waste products from the region.
- Modalities such as electric stimulation and ultrasound administered by a Physical Therapist.

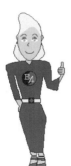

ERGELLATIP: IF YOUR SYMPTOMS PERSIST AFTER 2 DAYS, CONTACT YOUR DOCTOR OR MEDICAL PROFESSIONAL.

Avoid Neck Pain: Prevention

- Workstation ErgArrangement to minimize work stresses to the neck region.
- ErgErcises to stretch and strengthen the muscles of the neck and shoulder regions.

- Take regular breaks from the mouse and keyboard.
- Proper Posture. This includes modifying your posture about twice per hour.
- Avoid prolonged overhead activities.

Neck ErgErcises

<u>I. Warm Up</u>
Street Crosser

<u>Position:</u> **Sitting**
1. Allow your arms to rest comfortably by your side.
2. Slowly turn your head to the left until you feel a gentle stretch on the right side of your neck.
3. Slowly turn your head to the right until you feel a gentle stretch on the left side of your neck.

<u>Repetitions:</u> **10 times in each direction**

ErgleTip: THIS WARM UP IS MOST EFFECTIVE IF YOU RELAX YOUR SHOULDERS. MAKE SURE THAT YOU DON'T HOLD THEM UP BY YOUR EARS.

<u>Purpose:</u>
- Stretches the muscles on either side of your neck.
- Increases blood flow through the neck and head.
- Prevents:
    - Neck and arm pain.
    - Thoracic Outlet Syndrome.

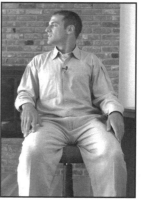

Left

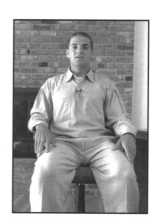

Center

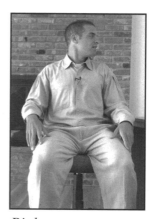

Right

II. Stretch
Puppy Dog

Position: Sitting

1. Place your head in the neutral position, looking straight ahead at your monitor.
2. Grab the bottom of the right side of your seat with your right hand.
3. Tilt your neck and head to the left side.
4. With your left hand, gently pull your head slightly further towards your left shoulder.

Hold position for: **10 seconds**

5. Release your left hand.
6. Slowly bring your head back to the starting position.

Repetitions: **5 times**

7. Repeat this ErgErcise to the right side.

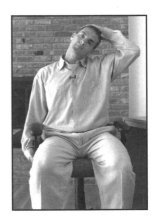

Puppy Dog (left)

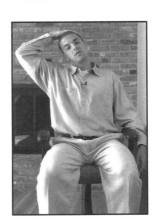

Puppy Dog (right)

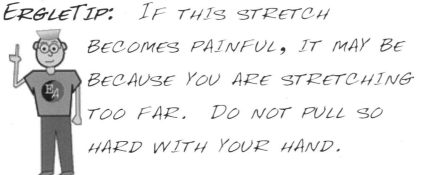

ERGLETIP: IF THIS STRETCH BECOMES PAINFUL, IT MAY BE BECAUSE YOU ARE STRETCHING TOO FAR. DO NOT PULL SO HARD WITH YOUR HAND.

Purpose:
- Stretches the muscles on either side of your neck.
- Increases blood flow through the neck and head.
- Prevents:
  - Neck and arm pain.
  - Thoracic Outlet Syndrome.

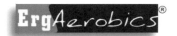

Muscle Pose Stretch

<u>Position:</u> **Sitting**

1. Place your head in the neutral position, looking straight ahead at your monitor.
2. Place your left hand on the back of your head.
3. Keeping your hand on your head, rotate your head half-way toward your left shoulder (45 degrees).
4. Keeping your back straight, gently pull your head towards your left knee.

<u>Hold position for:</u> **10 seconds**

<u>Repetitions:</u> **5 times**

5. Repeat this ErgErcise to your right side using your right hand.

<u>Purpose:</u>

- Stretches the levator scapula (muscles in the back of your neck that hold your head up).
- Increases blood flow through the neck and into and out of the head.
- Prevents neck and upper back pain.

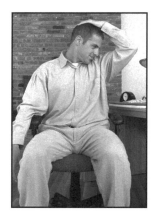

Muscle Pose (left)

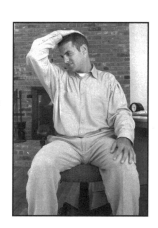

Muscle Pose (right)

<u>III. Strengthen</u>

Aye Caramba!!!

<u>Position:</u> **Sitting**

1. Place the palm of one hand on your forehead.
2. Hold your head completely still.
3. Try to push your head backward with your hand.
4. Do not allow your head to move.

<u>Hold position for:</u> **5 seconds**

<u>Repetitions:</u> **5 times**

<u>Purpose:</u>

- Strengthens the neck flexors (muscles in the front of the neck).
- Increases neck stability.
- Prevents:
    - Forward Head Posture
    - Thoracic Outlet Syndrome
    - Cervical Disc Herniations

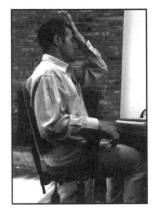

Aye Caramba!!!

Side Push

<u>Position:</u> **Sitting**

1. Place the palm of your left hand on the left side of your head, just above your ear.
2. Hold your head completely still.
3. Try to push your head to the right using your left hand.
4. Do not allow your head to move.

<u>Hold position for:</u> **5 seconds**

<u>Repetitions:</u> **5 times**

5. Repeat this ErgErcise to your right side, using your right hand.

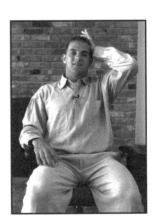

Side Push (left)

<u>Purpose:</u>

- Strengthens the muscles in the sides of the neck.
- Increases neck stability.
- Prevents Thoracic Outlet Syndrome.

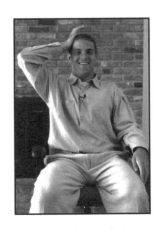

Side Push (right)

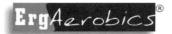

Wake Up!!!

<u>Position:</u> **Sitting**

1. Place both of your hands on the back of your head.
2. Hold your head completely still.
3. Try to push your head forward with both hands.
4. Do not allow your head to move.

<u>Hold position for:</u> **5 seconds**

<u>Repetitions:</u> **5 times**

<u>Purpose:</u>

- Strengthens the neck extensors (muscles in the back of the neck).
- Increases neck stability.
- Prevents:
    - Forward Head Posture.
    - Thoracic Outlet Syndrome.
    - Cervical Disc Herniations.

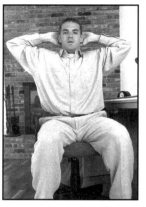

Wake Up!!!

Additional Neck ErgErcises

Egyptian (Chapter 5)
Tough Guy (Chapter 5)
Frankenstein (Chapter 5)

The Law of the JAW

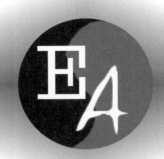

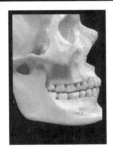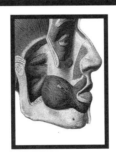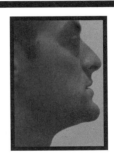

*E*rgle's computer monitor was always too far away from him. To see the screen better, Ergle, who is nearsighted, was constantly bringing his neck and head forward. This poor postural habit led to many problems with Ergle's jaw. He experienced headaches and pain in his jaw while sitting at his computer. Even worse, his jaw clicked when he ate, taking away the pleasures he normally associated with eating.

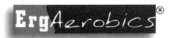

TMJ

- The temporomandibular joint (TMJ) is where the jaw bone (mandible) and the skull (temporal bone) meet.
- To feel the TMJ, place your finger in front of your ear and open and close your mouth.
- The condyle is the round head of the mandible, which inserts into the joint space (temporal fossa) near the front of the ear.
- Ideally, there is enough space at this joint during opening and closing of the mouth to allow for free movement of the condyle downward and out of the temporal fossa.
- A soft disc cushions the junction of these two bones and facilitates movement.

What is causing your TMJ pain?

TMJ Dysfunction

- TMJ Dysfunction occurs when the condyle does not move freely out of the fossa.
- The two jaw bones jam together when the mouth is opened or closed, causing pain.
- Pain may be in the form of:
    - Jaw pain
    - Headaches
    - Toothaches
    - Neck pain.

Symptoms of TMJ Dysfunction

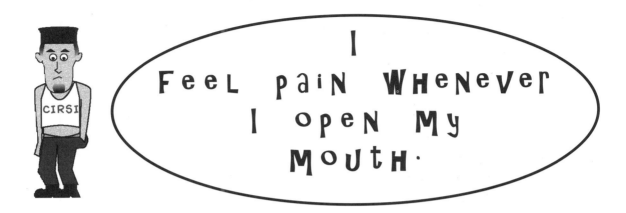

- Difficulty opening the mouth completely due to pain or locking of the jaw.
- Clicking or popping noises when opening and closing the mouth.
- Headaches, often recurrent and severe.
- Earaches accompanied by dizziness.
- Tenderness and swelling on the sides of the face.
- Toothaches that cannot be linked to nerve death, inflammation, or tooth decay.
- A burning, tingling sensation in the tongue, mouth, or throat.
- Neck and shoulder aches, with associated numbness in the arm and hands.

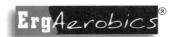

Who is @ risk for TMJ Dysfunction?

ERGELLAFACT: WOMEN ARE 4 TIMES MORE LIKELY THAN MEN TO EXPERIENCE TMJ DYSFUNCTION.

- People with poor postural habits. A Forward Head Posture causes the muscles around the jaw to tighten. The jaw gets pulled out of alignment, irritating the TMJ.

- People who breathe through the mouth. Breathing through your mouth leads to overuse and fatigue of the breathing muscles in the neck and upper chest. When fatigued, these muscles cannot help maintain proper posture and alignment. This results in a Forward Head Posture and subsequent TMJ irritation.

- People who talk on the phone for long periods of time with their head tilted to one side.

- People who have incurred a traumatic injury to the region, such as a direct blow to the jaw or a whiplash injury.

- People who habitually clench and grind their teeth due to stress or anxiety.

- People with an improper bite put undue strain on the muscles responsible for chewing.

ERGELLATIP: USE A HEADSET OR SIMILAR DEVICE TO HOLD YOUR PHONE WHEN TALKING FOR LONG PERIODS OF TIME.

Treatment of TMJ Dysfunction: Getting Better

- ErgErcise to stretch and strengthen neck and jaw muscles.
- Workstation ErgArrangement minimizes work-related stresses to the neck and jaw.
- Avoid or, at least, minimize painful activities.
- Improve posture to prevent Forward Head Posture.
- Apply ice to the jaw region for 10-minute intervals, 3 to 5 times per day, for the first 48 hours after experiencing pain.
- Massage area to flush out irritating waste products.
- Modalities, such as electric stimulation and ultrasound, administered by a Physical Therapist.
- Apply splints (provided by a dentist) over the teeth to keep the jaw from completely closing.

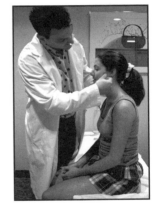

Physical Therapist performing a TMJ massage.

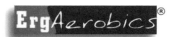

Avoid TMJ Dysfunction: Prevention

- Workstation ErgArrangement to minimize work-related stresses to the neck and jaw.
- ErgErcises to stretch and strengthen the muscles of the jaw.
- Take regular breaks from the mouse and keyboard.

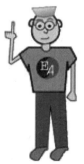

ErgleFact: THE WAY YOU POSTURE YOUR ENTIRE BODY WHILE WORKING AT A COMPUTER IS VITAL TO PREVENTING NECK, ARM, LEG, AND BACK CIRSIs.

- Maintain proper posture. This includes modifying your posture about twice per hour.
- Breathe with your mouth closed and your tongue touching the roof of your mouth.
- Relieve stress through regular exercise, meditation, etc.
- Avoid foods that are tough on the teeth and jaw.

Jaw ErgErcises

I. Warm Up
Big Mouth

Position: **Sitting**
1. Open and close your mouth.
2. Do not allow your jaw to shift to one side or the other.
3. Make this movement as smooth as possible.
Repetitions: **10 times**
Purpose:
- Increases circulation to the jaw muscles.
- Stretches the muscles used for chewing.
- Prevents TMJ Dysfunction.

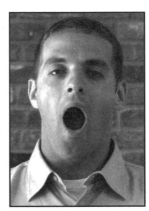

Big Mouth

II. Stretch
Jaw Breaker

Position: **Sitting**
1. Allow your mouth to hang partially open.
2. Shift your jaw to the right.
3. Shift your jaw to the left.
Repetitions: **10 times to each side**
Purpose:
- Stretches the jaw muscles. These muscles often tighten up when you maintain the same sitting or standing posture for long periods of time.
- Increases circulation to the jaw muscles.
- Prevents TMJ Dysfunction.

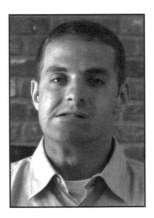

Jaw Breaker (right)

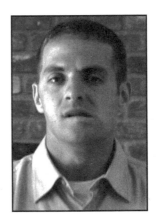

Jaw Breaker (left)

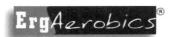

III. Strengthen

Biter

<u>Position:</u> **Sitting**

1. Close your mouth.
2. Place your tongue comfortably on the roof of your mouth.
3. Keeping your tongue on the roof of your mouth, lightly clench your teeth together.

<u>Hold position for:</u> **5 seconds**

<u>Repetitions:</u> **10 times**

<u>Purpose:</u>

- Strengthens the jaw muscles.
- Increases circulation to the jaw muscles.
- Prevents TMJ Dysfunction.

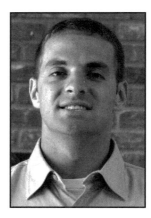

Biter

Additional Jaw ErgErcises

Street Crosser (Chapter 7)
Egyptian (Chapter 5)

THUMBS up

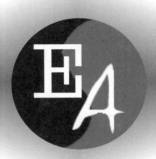

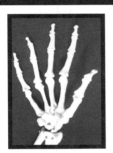 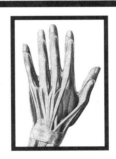 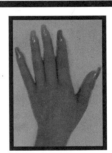

Throughout his youth, Ergle spent many hours playing computer games and typing on his keyboard. When playing the games, he used his thumb to press the joystick button. When typing, he used his thumb to tap the spacebar on the keyboard. Eventually, Ergle began feeling pain in his thumb, so he decided to give up playing video games. Ergle was confident that the pain in his thumb would go away. Despite his great sacrifice, Ergle continued to experience pain. This mystified our poor aching Ergle.

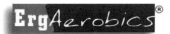

Thumb Region

- The abductor pollicis longus and extensor pollicis brevis are tendons that run from the wrist area to the fingernail side of the thumb.
- You can see and feel these tendons when you extend your thumb, as if you were hitchhiking.

What is causing pain in your Thumb?

DeQuervain's Disease

- This disease is a CIRSI of the thumb extensor tendons.
- Tapping the spacebar requires extension of the thumb.
- Continual keyboard tapping with your hands in their ordinary typing position causes repetitive stress on the thumb extensor tendons.
- Continual gripping activities with the wrist bent toward the pinkie can also cause DeQuervain's Disease.

Symptoms of DeQuervain's Disease

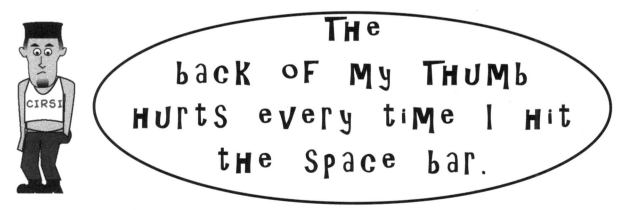

THe back oF My THUMb HUrtS every tiMe I Hit tHe Space bar.

- Pain in the thumb, wrist, and sometimes the forearm.
- Decreased thumb range of motion.
- Weak grip and pinch strength with the thumb.

Who is @ risk for DeQuervain's Disease?

- Computer users who continually tap the keyboard spacebar with their thumb.
- People who grip their pen tightly with their thumb while writing.
- Construction workers who hammer frequently.
- Fly fishermen who are constantly casting their fishing reel.

Treatment of DeQuervain's Disease: Getting Better

- ErgErcises to stretch and strengthen the muscles of the thumb and wrist.
- Workstation ErgArrangement to minimize work-related stresses to the thumb.
- Avoid or, at least, minimize painful activities.
- Improve posture to eliminate stress on the thumb.
- Apply ice to the region for 10-minute intervals, 3 to 5 times per day, for the first 48 hours after experiencing pain.
- Massage the area to flush out irritating waste products.
- Modalities, such as electric stimulation and ultrasound, administered by a Physical Therapist.
- Use of a brace to reduce stress at the thumb and wrist.

Avoid DeQuervain's Disease: Prevention

- Workstation ErgArrangement to minimize work-related stresses to the thumb and wrist regions.

- ErgErcises to stretch and strengthen the muscles of the thumb and wrist.
- Take regular breaks from the mouse and keyboard.
- Proper posture. This includes modifying your posture about twice per hour.
- Avoid tapping your computer keyboard spacebar with one thumb. Try to switch thumbs every hour.
- Avoid excessive pinching and gripping activities.

Thumb ErgErcises

I. Warm Up
The Sweep

Position: **Sitting**

1. Place your forearms on your armrests with your palms facing up.
2. Point each of your thumbs out to the side, away from your body.
3. Sweep your thumbs across your palms to where the pinkie meets the top of your palm.

Repetitions: **10 times**

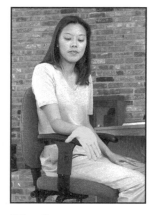 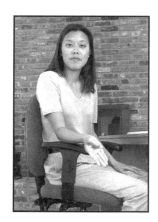 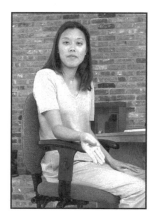

The Sweep

Purpose:
- Increases circulation to the thumb and hand.
- Prevents DeQuervain's Disease.

Bored Game

<u>Position:</u> **Sitting**

1. Place your forearms on your armrests with your palms facing each other.
2. Interlock your fingers.
3. Twiddle your thumbs forward.

<u>Repetitions:</u> **10 seconds**

4. Twiddle your thumbs backward.

<u>Repetitions:</u> **10 seconds**

<u>Purpose:</u>
- Increases circulation to the thumbs.
- Prevents DeQuervain's Disease.

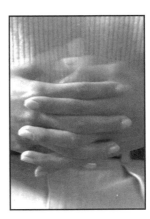

Bored Game

<u>II. Stretch</u>

Hammer Thumb

<u>Position:</u> **Sitting**

1. Place your forearms on your armrests with your palms facing each other.
2. Point your thumbs toward the ceiling.
3. Make a fist with each hand.
4. Tuck your thumbs into your fists and hold them firmly.
5. Tip your wrists forward as if slowly hammering a nail into a wall.

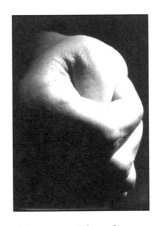

Hammer Thumb

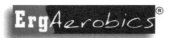

Hold position for: **10 seconds in the forward position**

Repetitions: **5 times**

Purpose:

- Stretches the thumb extensors and abductors (tendons that run along the top of your thumb from your wrist).
- Prevents DeQuervain's Disease.

III. Strengthen

The Push

Position: **Sitting**

1. Rest your forearms on your armrests.
2. Make a fist with your left hand.
3. Point your left thumb toward the ceiling.
4. Gently pull back on your left thumb with your right hand.
5. Resist by pushing with your thumb, not allowing your thumb to move.

Hold position for: **5 seconds**

Repetitions: **10 times**

6. Repeat with your right thumb, resisting with your left hand.

Purpose:

- Strengthens the thumb adductors and flexors (muscles that run along the palm side of your thumb).
- Prevents DeQuervain's Disease.

The Pull

Position: **Sitting**

1. Rest your forearms on your armrests.
2. Make a fist with your left hand.
3. Point your left thumb toward the ceiling.
4. Push forward on your left thumb with your right hand.
5. Resist by pulling with your thumb, not allowing your thumb to move.

Hold position for: **5 seconds**
Repetitions: **10 times**

6. Repeat with your right thumb, resisting with your left hand.

Purpose:

- Strengthens the thumb abductors and extensors (muscles that run along the top of your thumb from your wrist).
- Prevents DeQuervain's Disease.

It's all in the WRIST

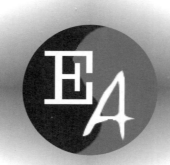

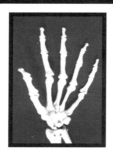 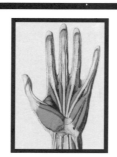 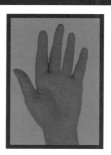

Ergle often typed for long periods of time without taking any rest breaks. When typing, Ergle's wrists were bent forward without support, and he maintained a Poor Posture. His hands cramped frequently, and he felt pain, tingling, and numbness in his thumb, index finger, and middle finger. Many of Ergle's coworkers doubted the sincerity of his complaints. Ergle could not figure out what the problem was, and so he fell deeper into the abyss of pain.

The Carpal Tunnel Region

- The wrist is the junction of the radius and ulna (the two forearm bones) and eight carpal bones (small bones of the hands).
- The carpal tunnel is at the base of the hand, on the palm side. It is the entryway of the median nerve and nine wrist flexor tendons through the wrist and into the hand.
- The median nerve provides sensation to the palm surface of the thumb, index finger, and middle finger. The sensation also extends to the thumb side of the ring finger, and around the nails of the same fingers.
- The median nerve stimulates muscles which help move the thumb, the index finger and the middle finger.

What is causing pain in your wrist and hand?

Carpal Tunnel Syndrome (CTS)

- Squeezing of the median nerve in the carpal tunnel. This occurs due to swelling of the median nerve and/or the tendons of the wrist.
- Most commonly, CTS is a CIRSI. This type of injury occurs from using a computer for hours on end with improper body mechanics and poor posture.
- The cumulative microtrauma from prolonged computer use causes the accumulation of irritating wastes, such as lactic acid, in the carpal tunnel region.
- Unless the user takes regular breaks and does some simple wrist ErgErcises, the waste products lead to swelling, and eventually, CTS.

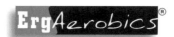

• Not all wrist pain is CTS. Other syndromes such as Herniated Cervical Disc, Thoracic Outlet Syndrome, and Shoulder Impingement are often misdiagnosed as CTS.

Symptoms of Carpal Tunnel Syndrome

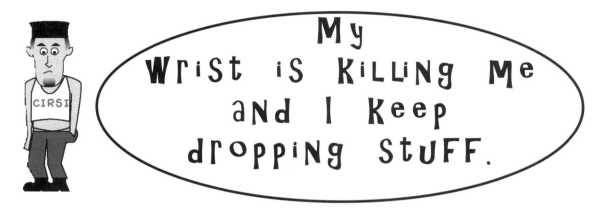

• Burning pain and tingling in the median nerve distribution (wrist, hand, thumb, and first three fingers).
• Deterioration of the muscles that move the thumb.
• Pain and numbness in the wrist and hand that interrupts sleep.
• Clumsiness and weakness of the affected hand.

Who is @ risk for Carpal Tunnel Syndrome?

• Computer users.
• People with occupations that involve repetitive wrist motions.
• Pregnant women, due to fluid retention and the general swelling of their joints.
• People of 50 years of age or older.
• Smokers, due to decreased circulation.

Treatment of Carpal Tunnel Syndrome: Getting Better

- ErgErcises to stretch and strengthen the muscles of the wrists and hands.
- Workstation ErgArrangement to minimize work stresses to the carpal tunnel region.
- Avoid, or at least, minimize painful activities.
- Postural improvement to eliminate stress from the wrist.
- Ice the region for 10 minute intervals 3-5 times per day for the first 48 hours after first experiencing pain.
- Massage in order to flush irritating waste products from the region.
- Modalities such as electric stimulation and ultrasound administered by a Physical Therapist.
- Wear a resting splint for the wrist at night. This prevents your wrists from bending forward and relieves pressure on the median nerve during sleep. This is a time when Carpal Tunnel Syndrome symptoms often flare up.

Avoid Carpal Tunnel Syndrome: Prevention

- Workstation ErgArrangement to minimize work stresses to the carpal tunnel region.
- ErgErcises to stretch and strengthen the muscles of the wrists and hands.
- Take regular breaks from the mouse and keyboard.
- Proper posture. This includes modifying your posture about twice per hour.
- Type with your wrists in a neutral position (not bent up or down).

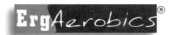

Wrist ErgErcises

<u>I. Warm Up</u>
Abra Cadabra

<u>Position:</u> **Sitting**

1. Rest your arms on your armrests with your wrists straight.
2. Face your palms toward the floor.
3. *Abra* = Slowly close your hands
4. *Cadabra* = Slowly open your hands.

<u>Repetitions:</u> **10 times**

<u>Purpose:</u>

- Increases blood flow to your hands.
- Relieves tension in the wrists and hands.
- Flushes waste products from the carpal tunnel region and the hands.
- Prevents Carpal Tunnel Syndrome.

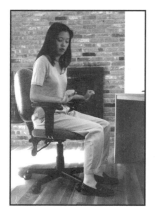

Abra

Cadabra

The Wave

<u>Position:</u> **Sitting**

1. Rest your forearms on your armrests, palms facing the floor.
2. Hang your hands over the ends of your armrests.
3. Lift your hands up slowly, as they will go comfortably.
4. Let your hands down slowly, as far as they will go comfortably.

<u>Repetitions:</u> **10 times in each direction**

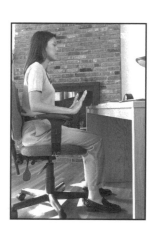

The Wave

Purpose:

- Increases blood flow to your hands.
- Relieves tension in the wrists and hands.
- Flushes waste products from the carpal tunnel region and the hands.
- Prevents Carpal Tunnel Syndrome.

Come Here

Position: **Sitting**

1. Rest your forearms on your armrests, palms facing the ceiling.
2. Hang your hands over the ends of your armrests.
3. Lift your hands up slowly, as far as they will go comfortably.
4. Let your hands down slowly, as far as they will go comfortably.

Repetitions: **10 times in each direction**

Purpose:

- Increases blood flow to your hands.
- Relieves tension in the wrists and hands.
- Flushes waste products from the carpal tunnel region and the hands.
- Prevents Carpal Tunnel Syndrome.

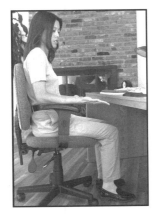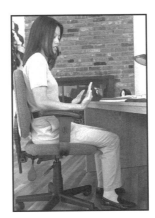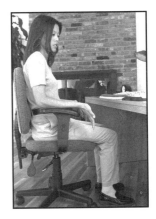

Come Here

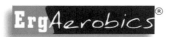

II. Stretch

Speak to the Hand

<u>Position:</u> **Sitting or Standing**

1. Straighten your left arm out in front of you, at shoulder height, as if pointing at something.
2. Bend your left wrist back so that your fingers point towards the ceiling.
3. With your right hand, gently pull back on your left hand fingers, bending your wrist back a little further.

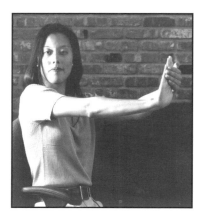

Speak to the Hand

<u>Hold position for:</u> **10 seconds**

<u>Repetitions:</u> **5 times**

4. Repeat with your right wrist, assisting with your left hand.

<u>Purpose:</u>

• Stretches the wrist flexors and finger flexors (muscles that run through the carpal tunnel and insert into the palm of the hand).
• Increases circulation throughout the wrists and hands.
• Prevents Carpal Tunnel Syndrome.

Screen Blocker

<u>Position:</u> **Sitting**

1. Move back from your monitor at least arms length.
2. Interlock your fingers in front of your chest.
3. Turn your palms away from your body.
4. Push your arms out in front of you.
5. Straightening your elbows.

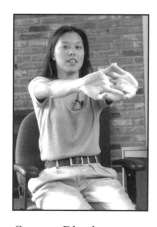

Screen Blocker

<u>Hold position for:</u> **10 seconds**

<u>Repetitions:</u> **5 times**

Purpose:

- Stretches the wrist flexors and finger flexors (muscles that run through the carpal tunnel and into the palm of the hand).
- Increases circulation throughout the wrists and hands.
- Prevents Carpal Tunnel Syndrome.

III. Strengthen

Desk Lift

Position: Sitting

1. Rest your forearms on your armrests.
2. Place your hands under your desk with your palms facing up.
3. Press the palms of your hands up against the underside of the desktop. Do not actually lift the desk, simply tighten the muscles in your forearm.

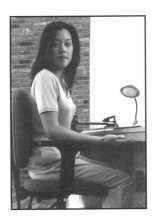

Desk Lift

ERGLETIP: DON'T PRESS TOO HARD. THE IDEA HERE IS TO ACTIVATE THE MUSCLES FOR STRENGTHENING PURPOSES.

Hold position for: **5 seconds**

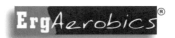

<u>Repetitions:</u> **5 times**

<u>Purpose:</u>

- Strengthens the wrist flexors (muscles running from your wrists up to the inner side of your elbows).
- Prevents Carpal Tunnel Syndrome.

ELBOW Room

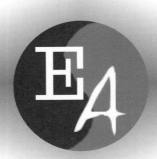

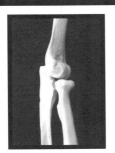 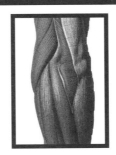 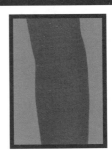

*E*rgle loves to play tennis and golf in his free time. But he recently began feeling pain on the outside of his elbow during and after playing tennis and on the inside of his elbow during and after playing golf. Ergle also works at his computer with his arms unsupported. This worsened his pain. Ergle decided the only way to heal the pain was to give up his favorite sports. But after several months, his elbow pain still persisted.

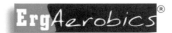

The Elbow Region

- The elbow joint is comprised of three bones. The humerus (upper arm) and the two forearm bones, the radius and the ulna.
- The wrist extensors (muscles that bend the wrist back) all originate at the lateral epicondyle. They all begin as the common extensor tendon and then branch out as they near the wrist.
- The extensor muscles work together during any activity involving grasping and picking up objects. In addition, the extensors are constantly holding your wrists up while you type.

What is causing pain in your Elbow?

Tennis Elbow

- Lateral Epicondylitis, or Tennis Elbow, occurs when the common extensor tendon becomes inflamed from repetitive use.
- Tennis Elbow is usually caused by stress placed on the common extensor tendon. This generally occurs from hitting a tennis backhand.
- At a computer workstation, the action of holding your wrists unsupported above a keyboard for prolonged periods causes continuous stress to be placed on the common extensor tendon. This eventually leads to Tennis Elbow.

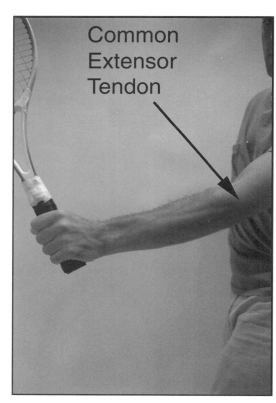

Common Extensor Tendon

Tennis Elbow

98

Symptoms of Tennis Elbow

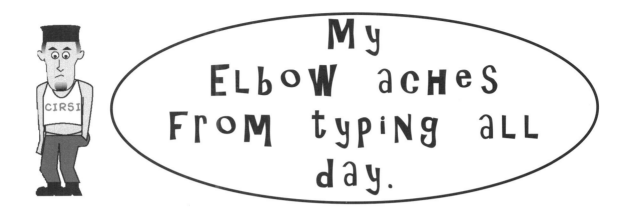

- Increased pain in the elbow after prolonged activity involving the wrist and hand.
- Stiffness in the elbow joint, with increased difficulty straightening the elbow.
- Tenderness when touching the lateral epicondyle.
- Pain when the wrist extensor muscles (top of forearm) are stretched.

Who is @ risk for Tennis Elbow?

- People with occupations involving repetitive use of the forearm musculature, including computer users, tennis players, and workers who carry and grip objects for prolonged periods of time.
- Computer users who type for long periods of time without supporting their arms on either their desk or an armrest.
- People 35 years of age and older. With age, muscle tendons become less flexible. This decreases their ability to tolerate everyday stresses, and therefore, increases the likelihood of tendon inflammation.

Treatment of Tennis Elbow: Getting Better

- ErgErcises to stretch and strengthen the muscles of the elbows and forearms.
- Workstation ErgArrangement to minimize work-related stresses to the elbow region.
- Avoid or, at least, minimize painful activities.
- Improve posture to eliminate stress from the wrist.
- Apply ice to the region for 10-minute intervals, 3 to 5 times per day, for 48 the first hours after experiencing pain.
- Massage area to flush out irritating waste products.
- Modalities, such as electric stimulation and ultrasound, administered by a Physical Therapist.
- Use of a brace to reduce stress at the elbow.

Avoid Tennis Elbow: Prevention

- Workstation ErgArrangement to minimize work-related stress to the elbow.
- ErgErcises to stretch and strengthen the muscles of the elbows and forearms.
- Take regular breaks from the mouse and keyboard.
- Proper posture. This includes modifying your posture about twice per hour.
- Avoid prolonged activity, such as typing or gripping heavy objects that overuse the forearm extensors.

Elbow ErgErcises

I. Warm Up
The Pump

Position: **Sitting**

1. Let your arms rest comfortably by your side.
2. Bend your elbows, bringing your hands up to your shoulders.
3. Straighten your elbows, bringing your hands back down to your sides.

Repetitions: **10 times**

Purpose:
- Increases blood flow to the entire arm.
- Prevents Tennis Elbow.

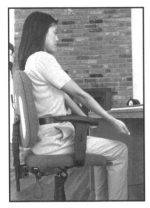 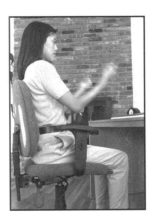 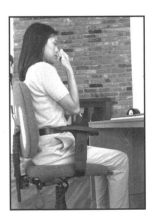

The Pump

II. Stretch
Pour Man's Stretch

Position: **Sitting or Standing**

1. Extend your left arm out in front of you, at shoulder height, as if you are pointing at something.
2. Make a fist and slightly bend your wrist downward.

3. Rotate your entire arm inward as if you are emptying a pitcher of liquid.

<u>Hold position for:</u> **10 seconds**

<u>Repetitions:</u> **5 times**

4. Repeat with your right hand.

<u>Purpose:</u>

- Stretches the wrist extensors (muscles from the outside of your elbow to the thumb side of your wrist).
- Prevents Tennis Elbow.

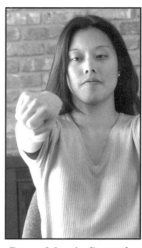

Pour Man's Stretch

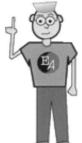

ERGLETIP: DO NOT BEND YOUR WRIST TOO FAR DOWN. THIS CAN CAUSE THE MUSCLES IN YOUR WRIST TO CRAMP.

Wrist Dip

<u>Position:</u> **Sitting or Standing**

1. Extend your left arm out in front of you, at shoulder height, as if you are pointing at something.
2. Bend your left wrist down so that your fingers are pointing toward the floor.
3. With your right hand, gently pull on the fingers of your left hand, bending your wrist down a little further.

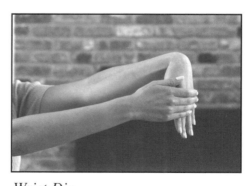

Wrist Dip

<u>Hold position for:</u> **10 seconds**

Repetitions: **5 times**

4. Repeat with your right hand, assisting with your left hand.

Purpose:

- Stretches the wrist extensors and finger extensors (muscles at the top of the wrist), which hold the hands up while typing or using a mouse.
- Increases the circulation throughout the wrists and hands.
- Counteracts the stresses on the wrists from working at a computer.
- Prevents:
    - Tennis Elbow
    - Carpal Tunnel Syndrome.

III. Strengthen

Reverse Desk Lift

Position: **Sitting**

1. Rest your forearms on your armrest.
2. Place your hands under your desk with your palms facing down.
3. Press the backs of your hands up against the underside of the desktop. Do not actually lift the desk, simply tighten the muscles in the back of your forearm.

Hold position for: **5 seconds**

Repetitions: **5 times**

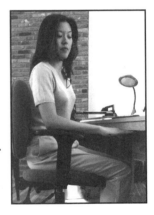

Reverse Desk Lift

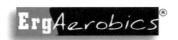

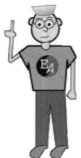

ErgleTip: Do not press too hard. The idea here is to activate the muscles for strengthening purposes.

Purpose:

- Strengthens the wrist extensors (muscles on the top of your wrists and along the top of your forearms).
- Provides opposition to the forces that allow Carpal Tunnel Syndrome to occur.
- Prevents Tennis Elbow.

SHOULDER the Load

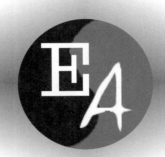

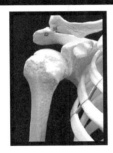 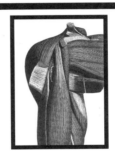 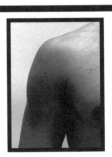

Due to his low self esteem, Ergle carried himself with a poor posture. Unlike the confident Ergella, who always stood tall and proud, Ergle would walk and sit with his shoulders rounded forward. Ergle did not realize the importance of a good posture, walking with his shoulders back, and carrying himself with pride. This postural habit eventually caused Ergle to experience pain in his shoulders.

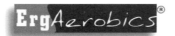

The Shoulder Region

- The glenohumeral joint, commonly known as the shoulder, is the area where the head of the humerus (top of the arm) and the glenoid fossa of the scapula (the socket of the shoulder) meet.
- The tendons of the supraspinatus muscle and biceps muscle run through this area.
- There is just enough space between the head of the humerus and the acromion (the tip of the shoulder) to allow for the passage of these tendons. This is known as the subacromial space.

What is causing your Shoulder pain?

Shoulder Impingement

- One of the most common injuries to the shoulder is a Shoulder Impingement.
- A Shoulder Impingement occurs when the tendons that glide through the subacromial space get squeezed or impinged between the head of the humerus and the acromion.
- An Impingement may occur if either the biceps or supraspinatus tendons become inflamed through overuse, or when poor posture limits the capacity for comfortable movement of the tendons through the subacromial space.
- Pain often occurs during forward elevation of the arm.

Symptoms of a Shoulder Impingement

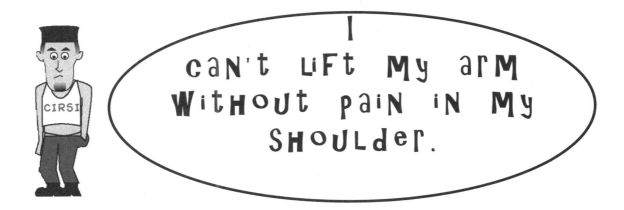

- Tenderness to the touch in areas where discomfort persists.
- Pain when lifting the arm above shoulder level.
- Pain and discomfort in the shoulder region.
- Pain in and stress to the shoulder after repeated movement or pro-longed activity.

Who is @ risk for a Shoulder Impingement?

- Computer users who repeatedly reach forward to use their computer keyboard or mouse.
- People who sit with a poor posture at a computer workstation. Sitting with Rounded Shoulders pinches the tendons that run through the shoulder region.
- Swimmers, window washers, or anyone else who performs activities involving excessive reaching above their head.

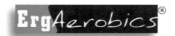

Treatment of a Shoulder Impingement: Getting Better

- ErgErcises to stretch and strengthen the muscles of the shoulders.
- Workstation ErgArrangement to minimize work-related stress at the shoulder.
- Avoid or, at least, minimize overhead activities.
- Improve posture to eliminate stress from the shoulder.
- Apply ice to the region for 10-minute intervals, 3 to 5 times per day, for the first 48 hours after experiencing pain.
- Massage the area to flush out irritating waste products.
- Modalities, such as electric stimulation and ultrasound, administered by a Physical Therapist.

Avoid Shoulder Pain: Prevention

- Workstation ErgArrangement to minimize work-related stress at the shoulder.
- ErgErcises to stretch and strengthen the shoulder muscles.
- Take regular breaks from the mouse and keyboard.
- Proper posture. This includes modifying your posture about twice per hour and avoiding Rounded Shoulders.

Shoulder ErgErcises

<u>I. Warm Up</u>
Pendulum

<u>Position:</u> **Standing with your right hip against your desk**

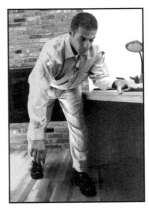

1. Bend forward and rest your right forearm and elbow on your desk.
2. Keep your back flat and look at the floor in front of you.
3. Allow your left arm to hang freely.
4. Slowly make clockwise circles with your left arm.

Pendulum

<u>Repetitions:</u> **10 times**

5. Reverse the action, making counterclockwise circles with your left arm.

<u>Repetitions:</u> **10 times**

6. Turn around and rest your left forearm and elbow on your desk.
7. Repeat with your right arm.

<u>Purpose:</u>
- Increases blood flow to the shoulder and arm.
- Stretches the rotator cuff (muscles that stabilize the arm in the shoulder socket).
- Relieves tightness and discomfort throughout the shoulder muscles.
- Prevents:
    - Pain and discomfort in the entire arm.
    - Shoulder Impingement Syndrome.

II. Stretch
Butterfly

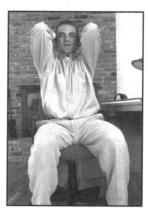

Butterfly

Position: **Sitting or Standing**

1. Interlock both of your hands behind your head, with your elbows out in front of you.
2. Slowly press your elbows back until you feel a slight pull in the front of your chest and shoulders.

Hold position for: **10 seconds**

Repetitions: **5 times**

Purpose:

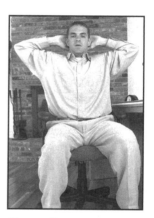

Butterfly

- Stretches the pectorals (chest muscles), which tend to tighten from sitting at a computer.
- Stretches the internal rotators (muscles of the shoulder that rotate the arm in toward the body).
- Increases blood flow to both arms.
- Prevents:
    - Shoulder Impingement Syndrome.
    - Thoracic Outlet Syndrome.

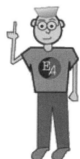

ERGLETIP: DO NOT PULL ON THE BACK OF YOUR HEAD. DOING SO CAN STRAIN THE MUSCLES IN THE BACK OF YOUR NECK.

Back Scratcher

<u>Position:</u> **Standing**

1. Bring both of your hands behind your back at belt level.
2. With your right hand, slowly pull your left hand up your back.
3. Hold your hands at a point where you feel a slight pull in your shoulder.

<u>Hold position for:</u> **10 seconds**

4. Slowly lower both hands.

<u>Repetitions:</u> **5 times**

5. Repeat with your right hand, assisting with your left hand.

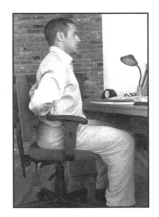

Back Scratcher

<u>Purpose:</u>
- Stretches the external rotator (muscles of the shoulder that rotate the arm away from the body).
- Increases blood flow to both arms.
- Prevents:
    - Shoulder Impingement Syndrome.
    - Thoracic Outlet Syndrome.

Additional Shoulder ErgErcises

Tough Guy (Chapter 5)
Frankenstein (Chapter 5)

Conclusion

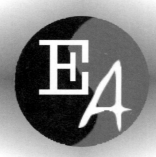

*F*ortunately for Ergle, Ergella introduced him to ErgAerobics, which has changed his life for the better. He now sits at his computer with a good posture, takes regular ErgErcise breaks, and uses proper ErgArrangement to minimize the stress placed on his body. At first, Ergle had to consciously remind himself to change his work habits. With time, however, they became second nature and a permanent part of his life. Ergle now lives a happy, pain-free life.

Cirsi Boy, on the other hand, continues to live in pain and refuses to do anything about it. He does not understand that it is never too late to change your work habits. Cirsi Boy has fallen into the abyss of pain and is unable to climb out. Like Cirsi Boy, many computer users refuse to make the changes necessary to prevent CIRSIs. Others simply do not know how to avoid the pain associated with working at a computer all day.

ErgAerobics provides you with the groundwork for preventing CIRSIs and improving your life. It is up to you to take the initiative. All you have to do is:

1. *ErgArrange your workstation.*
2. *Sit at your computer with a proper posture.*
3. *ErgErcise for at least one minute every hour.*

Frequently Asked Questions

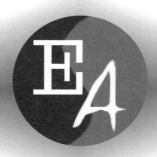

1. What is a CIRSI?

A CIRSI is a Computer Induced Repetitive Stress Injury, any injury resulting from the cumulative microtrauma of working at a computer.

2. What is ergonomics?

Ergonomics is the branch of science dealing with the interaction between man and machine. In the Computer Age, ergonomics most often refers to the set-up of a computer workstation. Ergonomics has become a garbage pail term referring to any product that is intended to relieve some of the physical stresses associated with working at a computer. So, an "ergonomic mouse" is one that helps prevent Carpal Tunnel Syndrome by supporting the wrist in a proper position for moving and clicking.

3. What is ErgAerobics?

ErgAerobics is a comprehensive CIRSI prevention system. This system has been designed as the solution to a $100 billion problem in the U.S. alone. ErgAerobics incorporates the most innovative ergonomic principles with preventative and rehabilitative exercises. In addition, readers are educated on behavior modification techniques essential to the prevention of CIRSIs.

4. Do ergonomic products prevent CIRSIs such as Carpal Tunnel Syndrome, Lower Back Pain, and Neck Pain?

Yes, many products on the market are helpful at preventing CIRSIs. However, even the best ergonomic keyboard will not automatically prevent Carpal Tunnel Syndrome. Behavior modification is an essential element in any injury prevention program. It is also necessary to incorporate proper computer workstation ErgArrangement, good sitting posture, taking regular rest breaks, and performing ErgErcises regularly.

5. Why do my hands hurt from typing at a computer?

Typing and using a mouse involve repetitive movement at the wrists and hands. During any repetitive movement there is an increased work demand on your muscles resulting in the accumulation of irritating waste products. After a period of constant work there is a resultant decreased blood supply to the muscles of your wrists and hands, causing them to cramp. This can eventually lead to Carpal Tunnel Syndrome.

6. How can I tell if I have Carpal Tunnel Syndrome?

A sure sign of Carpal Tunnel Syndrome is pain, tingling and numbness in the thumb, index and middle fingers of the hand. You will also experience weakness and swelling in the wrist and hand. If you experience these symptoms, you should consult your Physician or Physical Therapist.

7. I'm okay when I start work. As the day progresses, my wrists

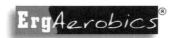

and hands start to swell. Why is that?

After typing all day, irritating waste products accumulate in the wrists and hands causing swelling to occur. Typically, the muscles of the wrists and hands get enough blood supply to get rid of the waste products that accumulate. However, the repetitive motion of typing all day decreases the amount of blood flow. This reduces the rate of repair, causing the wrists and hands to swell. It is important to take rest breaks and perform stretching ErgErcises. This allows the blood flow necessary for repair to return to the wrists and hands.

8. My job description is solely to sit in front of a computer and type all day. What can I do to avoid CIRSIs to my wrists and hands?

There are some jobs where repetitive motion at the wrist and hand is unavoidable. However, you can avoid injury by performing certain stretching and strengthening ErgErcises throughout the day which are neither time consuming nor conspicuous. These exercises will restore blood flow to the working muscles and are fully illustrated in the ErgErcise portion of this book.

9. Why does my thumb bother me when I tap the space bar on the computer keyboard?

By constantly tapping the space bar with your thumb you are stressing the tendons of the thumb which could cause De Quervain's Disease. Every hour you should switch the thumb you use to tap the space bar, allowing the tendons time to rest. For further information please read the section on De Quervain's Disease in the thumb chapter.

10. Is it important to have your arms properly supported while typing?

Your arms and hands get just enough blood supply to allow the muscles to work. Working with your arms unsupported against gravity will cause the muscles to demand a greater blood supply. Think of blood as fuel for your muscles. If you use up too much fuel early in the day, your muscles will run out of gas and fatigue. It is important to minimize the energy needed to work by providing upper extremity support while typing at a computer. A chair with armrests provides a sufficient amount of support. Tennis Elbow is one of many problems that can result from a lack of upper extremity support while typing.

11. My head and shoulders are usually slouched forward. Could this be the reason why I get neck and shoulder pain?

Forward Head Posture causes a decreased blood supply to the postural muscles of the neck resulting in a build up of irritating waste products. In effect, this posture increases the weight of the head on the postural muscles of the neck threefold. The postural muscles elongate, causing possible nerve impingement. Rounded Shoulders Posture compresses the tendons in the front of the shoulder, causing pain in the shoulder and arm.

12. I used to only have neck pain. Now I am experiencing pain down my arms. Why is this happening?

The nerves that exit the spine in the neck travel all the way down your arms to your fingertips. Any neck problems can result in subsequent pain down your arm. This is not a good sign. It is an indication that the symptoms are getting worse. You should consult your Physician or Physical Therapist.

13. I frequently experience headaches during and after working at my computer. Why does this occur?

Forward Head Posture will cause the postural muscles of your neck to tighten, potentially compressing the nerves that enter the head, causing pain. This poor postural habit can be the result of the computer monitor being placed too far away. As a result, the computer user moves their Head forward over their Neck to see the screen. Visual glare from a computer monitor can also cause headaches.

14. Is it okay to have my computer monitor off to my left side?

Having the monitor off to the left will cause the postural muscles on the left side of your Neck to tighten and on the right side to elongate. This muscular imbalance will eventually lead to difficulty turning your head to the right. Pain and discomfort may also result if a nerve impingement ensues.

15. If I maintain perfect posture all day will my aches and pains go away?

Even perfect posture is not good if it is maintained all day. Sustained posture, although perfect, will cause the postural muscles to fatigue. This is because the muscles never receive a break from posturing the body all day. If you sit all day, occasionally stand or adjust your chair or desk height slightly. This slight positional change will put different postural muscles to work, allowing others to rest.

16. Why is good posture important during work?

Good posture during work puts the least amount of stress on the working muscles and allows you to work longer with less fatigue.

17. I have the perfect chair to sit in, yet I still get muscle aches and pains. How should I sit while working?

The most perfect chair is useless if you do not sit in that chair properly. Always try to sit tall with a slight arc in your lower back and your chin tucked in. Do not slouch nor round your shoulders and head forward.

18. I just started sitting with better posture and my muscles now hurt. Why is this?

Do not be alarmed. Whenever muscles work in a different fashion it takes time for the specific muscles to adapt to a different work demand. Pain and soreness may occur initially. However, once the muscles get used to sitting with your improved posture the pain and soreness will go away.

19. What can I do to prevent my lower back from hurting after sitting for long periods of time?

Sustained sitting puts undo stress on the lower back. You should never sit for greater than one hour at a time. After each hour you should stand for a minute and perform Skywatcher ErgErcises. This ErgErcise will reverse the stress placed on the discs in the lower back during sitting.

20. I tend to slouch when I sit. Can this posture hurt my lower back?

Sitting, particularly for long periods applies a stress to the lower back. Slouching, which is a poor postural habit will only multiply that stress.

21. What is the best way to relax the muscles of my lower back after a long, hard day's work?

The least stressful position for the body is laying on your back with your hips and knees bent at a ninety degree angle. Lay on the floor with your calves and feet on the seat of a chair. This is a great way to reduce the stress of a long, hard day.

22. After looking at a computer screen my eyes start to hurt. What can I do to prevent this pain?

You can either place a protective screen over your monitor or periodically change the monitor angle to reduce glare.

23. Why is proper computer workstation set-up important for preventing work injuries?

Poor workstation design could cause undo stress to the working muscles. Studies have shown that approximately twenty percent of all computer workstation injuries are due to set-up. Please refer to Ergella's ErgArrangement Checklist for more information.

24. My body is not in any great pain after working at a computer for the last five years. Why should I change my work habits now?

Many injuries that develop at a computer are microtrauma injuries. This type of injury is the result of repeated small stresses over a period of time. Suddenly, the day comes when you're in a lot of pain. This type of injury is not like a broken arm or leg which happen suddenly. You might not feel any pain now but you could easily be on your way to a CIRSI. It is important to realize this and change your work habits now before it is too late.

25. Are exercises important during a work day?

If you take just sixty seconds every hour to perform some very simple stretching ErgErcises, the likelihood of you feeling pain at the end of the day greatly decreases. Exercise helps restore blood flow to working tissues, allowing the muscles greater endurance to perform the work at hand.

26. I don't have time to go to the gym. Are there any exercises I can perform at work?

Their are many stretching and strengthening ErgErcises you can perform at the computer workstation. These ErgErcises are not conspicuous nor time consuming and are fully illustrated in the ErgErcise portions of this book.

27. Is proper nutrition important to avoid aches and pains?

If you eat a proper diet your blood flow will be rich with the necessary vitamins, minerals and nutrients to help repair any damaged muscle. If your diet is filled with fatty foods the blood supply will no longer be like the supreme gas you fuel your car with. You will now be fueled by the cheap unleaded gas. Use the good stuff. It will improve the effectiveness and efficiency of your blood supply.

28. I smoke frequently. Can this affect the endurance of my muscles?

Smoking places poisonous carbon monoxide in your blood stream, decreasing the ability of your blood supply to provide your muscles with an adequate amount of necessary nutrients. Smoking also decreases the strength of the connective tissue in muscles, increasing the chance for muscle injury.

29. I find computer work very stressful. Can this be causing the muscle knots in my neck?

You could do absolutely nothing physical all day with the exception of thinking stressful thoughts and it is likely that you will obtain a muscle knot in your neck. Combine stress with working at a computer all day and you have big problems. Stress decreases the blood flow to your muscles causing irritating waste products to accumulate. If the stress is not stopped, the muscle has no time to rest and repair.

30. Why do my muscles occasionally go into muscle spasm?

A muscle spasm is a protective mechanism your body employs to prevent an injury from occurring. A spasm is caused by an insufficient blood

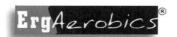

flow to the working muscles. It is your body's way of telling you to slow down or stop what you are doing in order to rest the muscle.

References

Anderson B. *Stretching*. Bolinas, Shelter Publications, Inc., 1980.

Apley AG, Solomon L. *Concise System of Orthopaedics and Fractures, ed 2*. London, Butterworth-Heinemann Ltd, 1994.

Bridger BS. *Introduction to Ergonomics*. New York, McGraw-Hill, 1995.

Caplan, D. *Back Trouble*. Gainesville, Triad Publishing Co., 1987.

Cunningham DJ. *Textbook of Anatomy*. New York, The MacMillan Company, 1902.

Dwight T, White JW, McMurrich JP, et al. *Human Anatomy, Sixth Edition*. Philadelphia, J.B. Lippincott, 1918.

Feiring J. *Textbook of Anatomy and Physiology, Sixth Edition*. Philadelphia, W.B. Saunders Company, 1939.

Grandjean E. *Ergonomics in Computerized Offices*. New York, Taylor & Francis, 1987.

Gray H. *Anatomy of the Human Body*. Philadelphia, Lea & Febiger, 1936.

Hebert, L. *The Neck Arm Hand Book*. Greenville, Impacc USA, 1989.

Hertling D, Kessler RM. *Management of Common Musculoskeletal Disorders: Physical Therapy Principles and Methods, ed 2.* Philadelphia, J.B. Lippincott, 1993.

Hoppenfeld, S. *Physical Examination of the Spine and Extremities.* Norwalk, Appleton and Lange, 1976.

Iglarsh ZA, Richardson JK. *Clinical Orthopaedic Physical Therapy.* Philadelphia, W.B. Saunders, 1994.

Kaplan AS. *The TMJ Book.* New York, Pharos Books, 1988.

Kisner C, Colby LA. *Therapeutic Exercise.* Philadelphia, F.A. Davis, 1990.

Lee K, Swanson N, Sauter S, et al. "A review of physical exercises recommended for VDT operators." *Applied Ergonomics.* 387-408, 23(6), 1992.

McKenzie, R. *Treat Your Own Back.* New Zealand, Spinal Publications Ltd., 1985.

Magee DJ. *Orthopedic Physical Assessment.* Philadelphia, W.B. Saunders, 1992.

Peterson B, Patten R. *The Ergonomic PC.* New York, McGraw-Hill, 1995.

Sobotta J, McMurrich JP. *Atlas of Human Anatomy.* New York, G.E. Stechert & Co., 1936.

White, AA III. *Your Aching Back*. Toronto, Bantam, 1983.

Index

About the Authors

Perry Bonomo, MAPT

Mr. Bonomo, age 31, has an MA degree in Physical Therapy and a BS in Health Sciences from Touro College. He currently co-owns a private physical therapy practice in New Milford, New Jersey and works for Marian Business Health Services in Sioux City, Iowa. He specializes in treating patients with CIRSIs and presents back school and neck/arm school classes to patients at the hospital. Mr. Bonomo is a member of the American Physical Therapy Association. He is certified at performing Functional Capacity Evaluations (FCEs) which are used to determine the level at which an injured worker is capable of returning to work and Work Site Analyses which determine risks in work design and worker habits that cause CIRSIs.

Daniel Seidler, MSPT

Mr. Seidler, age 29, is a member of the American Physical Therapy Association. He has an MS degree in Physical Therapy from Columbia University's School of Physicians and Surgeons and a BS in Marketing from the University of Vermont. He has been a physical therapist at the Albert Einstein Medical Center in Bronx, New York for three years. He is the director of the ergonomics and injury prevention program at the medical center.

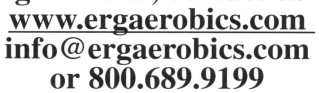
For other great CIRSI prevention products and services available from ErgAerobics, contact us @ www.ergaerobics.com info@ergaerobics.com or 800.689.9199

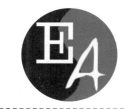

Order Form

Qty		Total
	ErgAerobics: Why does working @ my computer hurt so much? $14.95 each A comprehensive guide to prevent and treat Computer Induced Repetitive Stress Injuries. The book is easy to understand, educational, and entertaining.	
	The ErgErcise Video $14.95 each An instructional 25-minute video of 42 effective and inconspicuous ErgErcises that are easy to perform right at your workstation.The ErgErcise Video will teach you how to prepare your body for the computer revolution.	
	ErgAerobics Ergercise Poster $3.95 each An 11"X17" glossy with 8 essential ErgErcises.	
	Subtotal	
	Please add applicable sales tax	
	TOTAL	

<u>Payment Method</u>
___Check   ___Visa   ___Master Card   ___American Express
Credit Card #_____   Expiration Date___/___
Billing City and Zip_____
<u>Customer Information</u>
Name_____   E-mail_____
Address_____
City_____ State____ Zip_____ Phone# (____)_____-_____